Communication Disorders in Infants and Toddlers

Butterworth–Heinemann
Series in Communication Disorders
Charlena M. Seymour, Ph.D., Series Editor

Battle, D.E. *Communication Disorders in Multicultural Populations* (1993)

Battle, D.E. *Communication Disorders in Multicultural Populations, Second Edition* (1998)

Billeaud, F.P. *Communication Disorders in Infants and Toddlers: Assessment and Intervention* (1993)

Billeaud, F.P. *Communication Disorders in Infants and Toddlers: Assessment and Intervention, Second Edition* (1998)

Huntley, R.A. & Helfer, K.S. *Communication in Later Life* (1995)

Kricos, P.B. & Lesner, S.A. *Hearing Care for the Older Adult: Audiologic Rehabilitation* (1995)

Maxon, A.B. & Brackett, D. *The Hearing-Impaired Child: Infancy Through High School Years* (1992)

Velleman, S.L. *Making Phonology Functional: What Do I Do First?* (1998)

Wall, L.G. *Hearing for the Speech-Language Pathologist and Health Care Professional* (1995)

Wallace, G.L. *Adult Aphasia Rehabilitation* (1996)

Communication Disorders in Infants and Toddlers

Assessment and Intervention

Second Edition

Frances P. Billeaud, M.A., CCC-SLP
*Director of Clinical Activities, Department of Communicative
Disorders, University of Southwestern Louisiana, Lafayette*

Butterworth–Heinemann

Boston   Oxford   Johannesburg   Melbourne   New Delhi   Singapore

Butterworth–Heinemann supports the efforts of American Forests and the Global ReLeaf program in its campaign for the betterment of trees, forests, and our environment.

Library of Congress Cataloging-in-Publication Data
Billeaud, Frances P.
    Communication disorders in infants and toddlers: assessment and intervention/Frances P. Billeaud.—2nd ed.
        p.   cm.
    Includes bibliographical references and index.
    ISBN 0-7506-9952-3 (alk. paper)
    1. Communicative disorders in children. 2. Communicative disorders in infants. 3. Speech therapists—Practice. 4. Audiologists—Practice. I. Title.
        [DNLM: 1. Communicative Disorders—in infancy & childhood. 2. Communicative Disorders—diagnosis. 3. Communicative Disorders—therapy. WS 105.5.C8 B597c 1998]
    RJ496.C67B55   1988
    618.92'855--dc21
    DNLM/DLC
    for Library of Congress   97-43983
                                                                                                    CIP

British Library Cataloguing-in-Publication Data
A catalogue record for this book is available from the British Library.

The publisher offers special discounts on bulk orders of this book.
For information, please contact:
Manager of Special Sales
Butterworth–Heinemann
225 Wildwood Avenue
Woburn, MA 01801-2041
Tel: 781-904-2500
Fax: 781-904-2620

For information on all Butterworth–Heinemann publications available, contact our World Wide Web home page at: http://www.bh.com

10 9 8 7 6 5 4 3 2 1

Printed in the United States of America

6/2/99

Contents

Contributing Authors

Shalini Arehole, Ph.D., CCC-A
Associate Professor of Audiology, Department of Communicative Disorders, University of Southwestern Louisiana, Lafayette

Frances P. Billeaud, M.A., CCC-SLP
Director of Clinical Activities, Department of Communicative Disorders, University of Southwestern Louisiana, Lafayette

Thomas G. Rigo, Ph.D., CCC-A
Associate Professor of Audiology, Department of Communicative Disorders, University of Southwestern Louisiana, Lafayette

Suzanne Greenwood Thurmon, M.S., CCC-SLP
Former Director, Acadiana Early Intervention Program, Lafayette, Louisiana

Theodore F. Thurmon, M.D.
Professor of Pediatrics, Louisiana State University School of Medicine, Shreveport

Preface

Communication is the most complex of all human endeavors. Communicative competence is *the* basic academic skill—a fact so fundamental that it is seldom stated so explicitly. Similarly, the fact that air is necessary to sustain life is assumed to be universal knowledge and unnecessary to reiterate. The dramatic consequence of depriving an individual of air, however, draws immediate attention to itself and is attended to with heroic measures. In contrast, disorders of communicative development in young children are often overlooked—even by people who know there is (or suspect there may be) a problem. Despite the fact that delayed or disordered communication deprives the child of typical experiences during the period of optimal brain development, early intervention for atypical preverbal and early symbolic communicative development has only recently become an area of concern. Perhaps it is the complexity of the processes involved in developing communication competence that mitigates against actions that might be taken early on to address atypical communicative development.

Development of communicative competence begins before birth and is pivotal to cognitive, psychoemotional, behavioral, and social development. The ability to comprehend the communication of others (receptive ability), to then process one's own emotions and ideas and code the message one wishes to convey (mapping), and finally to convey that information to a communication partner (expressive ability) is communicative competence. Communication is achieved through a variety of means: gestures and body language, symbolic representations (e.g., the language system of the child's family or musical scores and mathematical formulas), and written symbols.

The earliest interactions between parent and infant set the stage for a child's linguistic and communicative development. Most babies begin using words meaningfully by the end of the first year of life and rapidly build a repertoire of spoken words—and an even larger repertoire of words they understand. During the first years of life, most children master the essentials of oral language: basic phonology, semantics, morphology, syntax, and pragmatics. By age 3, children are usually quite adept at relating their feelings and experiences and in conversing with others. By this time, we expect the typical child to be reasonably intelligible to most listeners.

The development of communicative competence depends on a range of basic factors, all of which interact with and have the capacity to influence each of the other factors. Between 6% and 10% of infants born each year fail to follow the typical course of language development as a result of some disturbance in the synergistic relationships among the basic elements that promote developmental processes. At any given time in the United States, there are 630,000–1,050,000 infants and toddlers in the birth-to-36-month age group who are experiencing significant problems with communicative development that affect their social, emotional, behavioral, and preacademic abilities.

Atypical communicative development may be associated with a wide range of causes and perpetuating factors, the nature, seriousness, and timing of which affect the prognosis for a favorable outcome. Sometimes the communicative problem is the sole area of a child's developmental difficulty; sometimes the communicative problem is one of a complex of problems that affect physical growth, cognitive and motor functions, and other areas of development.

Since publication of the first edition of this work in 1993, a great deal of research across a range of professional disciplines has been generated in the area of communicative development and disorders. This interdisciplinary knowledge base has improved our ability to predict which risk factors are associated with atypical communicative development and to identify, assess, diagnose, and manage communicative problems in the infant-toddler population. Significant progress has been made in technology and pharmacology for sustaining the lives of smaller and smaller premature babies and infants born with a variety of medical conditions and sensory impairments. Knowledge of management techniques for infants in the preverbal stages of development who are experiencing an array of perplexing delays and disorders has mushroomed. Simultaneously, many changes have occurred in the area of health care delivery systems, with managed care emerging as a "megaforce" that affects all areas of professional activities for communicative disorders specialists, as well as their colleagues in related professions: pediatrics, social work, nursing, occupational therapy, physical therapy, early childhood education, and medical subspecialties that deal with infant-toddler health and development.

The first legal rulings in challenges to early intervention management policies and practices have emerged and continue to be promulgated across the nation. As of this writing, the rules and regulations governing the implementation of the 1997 reauthorization of the Individuals with Disabilities Education Act (IDEA) are yet to be developed, placing funding of some programs at risk and causing a significant degree of frustration among practitioners who must deal with the immediate needs of babies and families while governing regulations and policies of existing systems are in flux.

This book is intended for communicative disorders specialists who are interested in serving the youngest group within the pediatric population. It is meant to be a clinical reference tool for professionals and a guide to practical resources applicable to working with children diagnosed with or at risk for communicative delays or impairments. Because a great deal of the work done in this area involves working with families and peer professionals in related fields, an effort has been made to provide information about the processes of teaming, referral, collaboration, and communicating efficiently and effectively with others in the face of the demands placed on the system by the forces of managed care. It may also serve as a resource for preservice training programs in their endeavor to address the needs of the communicatively impaired across the life span.

This edition of *Communication Disorders in Infants and Toddlers: Assessment and Intervention* supplements the content of the first edition with new information throughout. Two new chapters have been added: one on heritable disorders and another on habilitation of hearing-impaired infants and toddlers. The glossary and appendices have been expanded as well. An effort has been made to distill findings and information reported in the research literature from a variety of professional disciplines. Although a volume of this scope can only sample such studies, references are provided for further study. A list of pertinent organizations also has been included. As in the first edition, and as is frequently the case in the discipline, the terms *communication* and *communicative* are used interchangably throughout the text.

A special note of appreciation goes to the contributing authors: pediatrician and medical geneticist Theodore F. Thurmon; Suzanne Greenwood Thurmon, former director of one of the first early intervention centers in the country; and audiologists and university colleagues Thomas G. Rigo and Shalini Arehole. My thanks are extended to all of the individuals and groups who have contributed their time so generously and have shared their expertise to make this new edition a reality. It is our sincere hope that readers will find this work to be a useful tool In acting out their dedication to the families and babies in need of special care and understanding. Their welfare is our common bond.

FPB

1

Communication Impairment in Infants and Toddlers: A Frame of Reference

Frances P. Billeaud

This book is about people and their relationships. It is about parents and families whose babies are different. It is also about men and women who come into the lives of these families because of their children's atypical development.

This book is packed with data about conditions that result in communication disorders and about the system of care available to affected children and their families. There is information about treatment and intervention strategies, research, and technology. Mere possession of knowledge and technical exper tise, however, is not enough. Ultimately, the professionals' knowledge, skills, and competencies are only effective to the extent they are applied for the benefit of individual children and their families in specific circumstances.

This book is about challenges and hopes. It is also about facts that are hard to hear and hard to deliver. It is about interactions with professional peers, babies, and families. It is about real people like those whose stories follow.

Ellen

"There's something wrong with my child," Ellen's mother told the pediatrician. She was assured that her fear was unfounded. As the mother of 3-month-old Ellen, Ann was told that she was expecting too much too soon of her beautiful little daughter. Ellen's constant crying and infrequent periods of sleep were ascribed to "just a little colic," possibly complicated by transmission of her mother's anxieties during caregiving activities. The pediatrician assured Ann that once Ann herself could get a little more sleep and relax and enjoy the baby, Ellen would settle down too. Over the next several months, the doctor reassured Ann that everything was normal, despite Ann's repeated assertions that something was wrong. The doctor pointed to the child's continued weight gain, her normal head circumference, blood-test results, and other physical evidence that Ellen met expectations for development.

By the time Ellen was 15 months old, she was still not sleeping well. She had frequent bouts with ear infections. She frequently cried for hours at a

1

time. Although she was sitting up, she tended to wobble. She was not walking, and she did not talk. She drooled constantly. Ann was exhausted. She was also frustrated; it seemed that no one would take her fears about Ellen's development seriously. Ann's husband Roger was concerned too, but his business had not been going well, and he was spending all of his time trying to avoid losing it. In desperation, Ann begged the doctor to refer Ellen to a pediatric neurologist in a nearby town. He agreed that it was time to look into Ellen's problems with walking and talking. Six weeks later (the earliest appointment that could be arranged) Ann drove the 80 miles to keep Ellen's 10:00 AM appointment with the neurologist. By noon, Ann had the diagnosis: Ellen had cerebral palsy.

David

At 36 months of age, David was an active little fellow who loved playing with his collection of toy trucks. He was a bit of a picky eater, but his mother found it easy to please him with the few foods he enjoyed eating—pizza, french fries, and fish sticks. He was not impressed when his baby sister arrived. The family was pleased that the new baby did not have the feeding problems David had in the early months: David was hospitalized once because he became so dehydrated. After the mother's difficult delivery with David, it seemed ages before he was finally healthy. However, once he was able to keep food down, he grew and developed. David's father, Henry, was in his final year of medical school. It was fortunate that David's early medical problems received prompt attention thanks to Henry's connections at the teaching hospital. It was also fortunate that the family's finances allowed Victoria, David's mother, to be at home with the children on a full-time basis.

Victoria quizzed Henry about why David's speech was so slow in developing. He was saying three or four words, but he did not use them often. When he used them, they were very hard to understand—sometimes his few words were not even pronounced the same way from one utterance to the next. Henry arranged to have David's hearing tested at the hospital. The results indicated no problem, ruling out the most likely cause of the scant speech development. Victoria knew there was some logical explanation and urged Henry to check the resources in the medical library. He did not find any leads there, but he promised to keep trying, although he knew his schedule did not allow much time for personal research.

It was obvious to everyone in the family that David was intelligent. He was adept at constructing elaborate structures with his blocks. He seemed to understand everything that was said to him. He was intrigued with his grandfather's farm equipment and had learned to identify many different types of trucks and farm implements, easily choosing the right one from the array of pictures in his favorite book when asked to do so.

It was true that David's attention span was brief, but he seemed interested in so many different things, and he *was* able to sit down with his dad to look at books for 15–20 minutes when Henry had time to play with his son. David especially liked sitting in Henry's lap, supported snugly against his dad's warm chest and surrounded by his big arms as they looked at pictures of combines, reapers, dump trucks, and highway tankers. Henry was especially proud that David liked this particular activity, because David usually rebuffed his parents' and grandparents' attempts to offer affectionate little pats and strokes.

Victoria finally convinced Henry that a speech-language pathologist (SLP) might be able to tell them something they could do to help David talk more. An SLP from the nearby university, a friend of the SLP at the hospital, agreed to go to the house to see David in surroundings that were familiar to him, where he had access to his toys. The SLP found David to be quite active, just as his mother had described when the appointment had been set up by phone. He was cooperative, bringing requested items to the SLP for inspection, opening his mouth willingly to allow a view of the oral mechanism, and offering the visitor a cookie before drinking apple juice from his covered cup. The SLP noticed that the sipping flange of the plastic cup had obviously been chewed. Victoria explained that David seemed to need to "bite down on the cup" to swallow liquids. She guessed it was the result of taking his bottle away before the baby came. When Victoria tried to give him juice from an open-top cup or tumbler, he "always got too much at one time" and choked. Victoria added that he also liked to "suck on his food," often discarding portions of it, such as toppings other than cheese on the pizza. After observing David in several activities, the SLP asked Victoria to take David to the university's speech and hearing clinic for further evaluation. The SLP disclosed that she suspected the child had oral-motor coordination problems that could be directly related to his difficulty in producing speech. That diagnosis was subsequently confirmed. David now continues to receive speech therapy from a private practitioner in the city where his father is the newest member of the medical community.

Kent

Kent's mother and father describe him as "all boy." He is the younger of two children born to Courtney and Michael. Kent's sister is 3 years older and is in first grade. Michael is an engineer. Courtney quit her job when Kent was born to become a full-time mom. She would like to return to work, at least part time, now that Kent is 3 years old, but she has been unable to locate a daycare center willing to take him. He is unusually handsome and loves playing outdoors. He is not yet fully toilet trained and does not talk much. Courtney worries about his speech, because the times he has spoken have been few and far between. Words she has heard him use seem to have disappeared, almost as if "he said them once and then lost interest in doing it again." His sister's friends have begun asking questions about why Kent doesn't talk and why he "acts funny." She just laughs and responds, "That's just how boys are." But she knows there must be something else and wonders why Kent doesn't play with her or use his toys "the right way."

Courtney describes Kent as affectionate "when he wants to be," checking frequently to be sure she is nearby, but not responsive to her cuddling, which his sister loved when she was his age. Kent seems unable to concentrate on most things but is "able to totally immerse himself in a cartoon or action show on TV." His mother and father agree that he is "the most stubborn child" they know when he does not want to do something, even when it is something as simple as getting dressed in the morning or turning off the TV set.

Michael and Courtney know that they have to watch carefully what Kent eats because he has allergies to many cereal grains. Foods that contain even small amounts of corn sweetener or many other cereal products cause him to have stomachaches and set off extreme hyperactivity, sometimes lasting far into the night and requiring one parent or the other to remain awake to prevent the child from going outside "to run off his energy."

Because Kent does not always respond to requests or comply with directions, Michael and Courtney fear that the child will be viewed as "retarded." They point out that he is quite intelligent "in his own way." They are aware that his lack of social interaction and speech will cause problems in school when the time comes, and they would like to enroll him in a program for children with delayed onset of speech. However, when they visited the program, they were alarmed to see that some of the children had strange behaviors. The other children did not seem to pay much attention to each other or their surroundings, and Kent's parents were afraid Kent might pick up "some bad habits" by watching them. The teacher told them that Kent would have to be tested to be sure that he was eligible for enrollment in the program. They were sure that Kent "could not cooperate" well enough to be tested and feared that he might be "labeled" if they gave their permission to try. They were emotionally torn and frustrated by the seemingly limited avenues open to them.

Cedric

Ruby's teenage daughter ran away from home only 2 weeks after giving birth to Cedric, a full-term, healthy, beautiful little boy. Cedric is 4 years old, and Ruby is the only mother he has ever known. She is proud of Cedric. On the days Ruby works, he stays with a neighbor who cares for two other children in her home. The babysitter brags that Cedric is the best child she has ever looked after. He is polite and bright, helping his grandmother with household chores, keeping his room neat, and even helping the sitter care for the two younger children when he is there. Although Cedric is eligible to attend Head Start, Ruby feels that he will have plenty of time to "be in school" and prefers having him in a child care setting with which she is familiar. Ruby's one concern is that Cedric has never talked. He does communicate, however, in a very lively way. His eyes dance when he is excited, his facial expressions are captivating, and he has an extensive repertoire of gestures that help him get his points across. It is almost as if he does not really need to talk.

When Ruby took Cedric to the university speech and hearing clinic, she did so only because the babysitter suggested that it would be a good idea to "have him checked out before school starts." As a standard part of the communication evaluation, a hearing test was administered. The audiologist, who suspected that the child probably had a hearing loss, was startled to find that Cedric had a profound bilateral sensorineural hearing loss. When Ruby was told of this, she vehemently denied that it could be true. She insisted on "showing" the staff how well Cedric could hear. Because she was so agitated, the staff agreed to let her demonstrate her point and watched through a one-way mirror as she gave Cedric directions (which he followed with ease), made requests of him (with which he readily complied), and responded to his spontaneous and elaborate nonverbal communication efforts.

Satisfied that she had proven to the staff that Cedric could, indeed, hear despite what the "machines" said, Ruby emerged from the observation room all smiles. When she was asked to allow an examiner to go into the room with Cedric while she watched and listened from the other side of the one-way mirror, she readily agreed. Once again, Cedric responded to the adult's bids for communicative interaction. However, when the examiner turned her back on Cedric and made requests, he continued playing with the toys without responding. Ruby was embarrassed that Cedric was being uncharacteristically "rude" to the examiner. When it was pointed out that Cedric could not see her face when she spoke, Ruby insisted that it ought not to make a difference. The staff member sitting with Ruby offered to let her use the intercom microphone to communicate with Cedric. She accepted the offer and began giving specific directions to the child: Cedric did not respond at all. She attempted several times to get his attention but could not. When the examiner in the room with him stated that she thought Cedric was an exceptional speechreader but did not hear what she was saying, Ruby dissolved in tears, acknowledging Cedric's hearing impairment for the first time.

Bitsy

She was nicknamed Bitsy because her real name—Elizabeth—seemed far too big for the tiny premature child lying in the neonatal intensive care unit (NICU). She would be going home in a few days if everything continued to go well. The NICU was the only home she had known since her birth 2 months ago. Although she weighed less than 4 pounds at birth, the main worry was her cleft palate and cleft lip, which interfered with her ability to get sufficient nutrition when she was strong enough to be taken off nasogastric feedings. The nurses said she had to be watched carefully because she sometimes forgot to breathe. Bitsy's mom, Karen, had learned a lot from the nurses about caring for her, and she felt fairly comfortable feeding her with them nearby to help in case anything went wrong. Bitsy's head had to be supported while she was positioned upright during feedings so that she would not choke. A special bottle and nipple had to be used because her sucking was not normal. After the surgeries to close Bitsy's lip and palate, the nurses said she would do much better with her feedings. Karen was excited about taking Bitsy home to her new room with the ruffled curtains and freshly painted bassinet, but she was also scared. There was so much to do just to take care of Bitsy. Karen caught herself daydreaming about Bitsy's future: How would she sound when she started to talk? Would other people be able to understand her? Would she have a scar on her face that would cause her embarrassment, especially when she reached her teenage years? Karen had only known one other person who was born with a cleft lip and palate, her mother's older cousin, and her speech was very nasal. Who could help her teach Bitsy how to talk so that she didn't have that kind of speech? Karen was stirred from her daydreaming when Bitsy coughed.

FAMILIES AS FIGURES IN THE EPIDEMIOLOGIC DATABASE

Ellen, David, Kent, Cedric, and Bitsy are parts of an epidemiologic database; however, first and foremost they are children with caring families whose concern for their welfare is obvious. Some of these families learned of their child's communication problems early, and others learned later. Some had to deal with other, sometimes life-threatening, issues before turning their attention to the communication difficulties. In each case, the impact of the child's communication disorder is far reaching and affects the entire family unit. The hopes, dreams, and expectations of the families of these children have been altered in significant ways by the existence of the child's communicative difficulties.

Statistical Overview

Accurate statistical data on the number of children affected by communicative disorders in this country is difficult to obtain for many reasons. The primary reason is the variability in categories of reporting used by different governmental agencies and by different professional groups that view the population from different perspectives. As the Assistant Secretary for Planning and Evaluation of the U.S. Department of Health and Human Services pointed out,[1] "Few data sources exist on children with disabilities and estimates vary by how disability is defined. . . . In December 1992, 548,700 children under 18 received SSI [Supplementary Social Security Income], which provides cash assistance to certain low-income children with disabilities" (p. 1). By way of contrast, the U.S. Department of Education[2] reported that a total of 3,507,488 children in the 6- to 21-year age group received special education services in categories of disability usually served by communicative disorders specialists (i.e., hearing impairment, speech-language impairment, multiple disabilities, and specific learning disabilities). On the other hand, agencies that track prevalence and incidence figures relevant to public health often use categories related to childhood chronic illness and use different criteria to define disability or impairment of function resulting from those categories. Newacheck and Taylor[3] (p. 364) summarized methodological problems in identifying affected populations, which are spawned by the definitional variations and frustrate the effort to arrive at reliable figures:

> Partly because . . . common definitional criteria are lacking, the research community has generated widely differing estimates of the prevalence of childhood chronic conditions. Additional variation results from the different methods used in collecting prevalence data [studies based on population, clinical studies, parental reports, medical records review, types of conditions reported]. As a result of these different methods, published estimates of the proportion of children with one or more chronic illnesses range from less than 5% to more than 30%.

To complicate the issue, the term *disability* is defined differently by policy makers in dealing with issues of education and those dealing in issues of health. The 1992 National Health Interview Survey, conducted by the Census Bureau for the National Center for Health Statistics, used a household survey to survey the noninstitutionalized U.S. population. In that study, *disability* was broadly defined to include "any limitation in activity due to a chronic health condition or impairment."[4] For children under 5 years of age, whose ability to engage in play was used as the gauge of disability, 2% were reported to have been so affected. The criterion for disability in this study changed (from ability to engage in play to ability to attend school) for children between 5 and 17 years of age, making comparisons among age groups difficult at best. Some social service and health tracking systems define disability in terms of a condition or set of conditions that interfere with activities of daily living.

The 1991–1992 Survey of Income and Program Participation collected information about chronic conditions, including functional limitations related to those conditions using the extended International Classification of Impairments, Disabilities, and Handicaps that encompasses the personal and social consequences of diseases. "For children aged 0–5 years, disability was defined as (1) limitation in the usual kind of activities done by most children the same age or (2) receipt of therapy or diagnostic services by the child for developmental needs. For children over 6 years, disability was any limitation in the ability to do regular school work"[5] (p. 1).

According to Wenger and colleagues,[4] 5 million conditions cause disabilities among 4 million children, an average of 1.2 conditions per child. The fifth most common group of disabling conditions among children in the National Health Interview Survey was "speech impairments," which affect 335,000 or

6.7% of children under 18 years of age. Statistics cited in this survey for other groups often served by communicative disorders specialists included an additional 190,000 (3.8%) children under 18 years of age with hearing impairments, 167,000 (3.4%) with learning disabilities, 108,000 (2.2%) with congenital anomalies, and 99,000 (2%) with cerebral palsy.

Diagnostic Classifications

To further confound the difficulty of obtaining accurate epidemiologic data, diagnostic classifications count some children more than once and others not at all. Consider the difficulty of comparing children who have some or many labels that cross the boundaries among specific medical diagnostic categories listed in *Current Procedural Terminology*[6] and *International Classification of Diseases*[7] used by physicians, the American Academy of Pediatrics' *Classification of Child and Adolescent Mental Diagnoses in Primary Care*,[8] the codes for psychological and psychiatric diagnoses outlined in the *Diagnostic and Statistical Manual* of the American Psychiatric Association,[9] the *Diagnostic Classification of Mental Health and Developmental Disorders of Infancy and Early Childhood*,[10] Individuals with Disabilities Education Act (IDEA) educational eligibility guidelines (which vary from state to state for infant, toddler, and family services covered under Part H/Part C),[11] and various state guidelines for services under Section 504 of the Rehabilitation Act of 1973.[12]

Whatever the actual figures may be, the U.S. Department of Education recognizes that the number of infants and toddlers receiving services under Part H/Part C of IDEA is below expectations in terms of reaching children who are eligible because of diagnosed medical conditions, documented developmental delays, or both. The federal government is urging states to find and provide services to all eligible children.[13] At the same time, professionals in early intervention are pleading with their colleagues to help children with "less severe disabilities" who often go untreated (and sometimes unrecognized by parents and professionals) until 5–8 years of age.[14]

PRACTICAL APPROACHES TO FRAMING THE ISSUES

In the short time between birth and the third birthday, most children progress from being 100% reliant on others to recognize and respond to their needs to being individuals capable of moving about in familiar surroundings, thinking about their experiences, comprehending what is being said to them, and using speech with a reasonable level of intelligibility to share their feelings and intentions. Those important milestones are the outcomes of typical or "normal" child development and emerge from a broad range of interdependent variables, each of which is capable of affecting the others. Table 1.1 is a condensed display of elements contributing to communicative development.

Table 1.1 Elements Affecting Early Language Development*

Neurophysiologic factors	Early language sequences	Synergistic "demands"	Developmental domains
Regulatory capacity	Perception of stimuli	Sensory integration	Sensory integration
Sensory integrity	Memory for experiences	Phonation dynamics	Physical growth
Brain structure integrity	Presymbolic (R) (e.g., sound discrimination)	Resonation dynamics	Gross- and fine-motor control
Myelination process	Presymbolic (E) (e.g., babbling, vocal play)	Articulation dynamics	Emotional adjustment
Cortical integrity	Symbolic, nonverbal (E, R)	Gross- and fine-motor control	Cognitive skills
Physical health	Communication skills	Cognitive processing	Social skills
Emotional and environmental factors	Symbolic, nonvocal (E, R) (e.g., gestures, "baby signs")	Executive function (e.g., intonation, stress)	Communication skills
Attachment and emotional security	Symbolic, first words and holophrasis (E)	Integration of social and cultural conventions	
Experiential exposure	Symbolic complexity (E, R) (e.g., semantics, syntax, and morphology)		
Need and motivation to communicate			
Opportunity to communicate			
Impact of effort to communicate (i.e., choices, rewards, and power to affect others or the environment)			

E = expressive modality; R = receptive modality.
*Language development, both typical and atypical, occurs in conjunction with simultaneous maturation and development across many parameters. Anything that disturbs development in one area has the potential to affect development in other areas (transactional theory of development).

Transactional Factors in Development

Hallett and Proctor[15] pointed out the interdependency of biological structures, maturation of the central nervous system, and environmental processes on the developing child:

> By the second or third year of extrauterine life (with brain weight reaching 80% of adult weight), the cerebral cortex begins to approach the metabolic rate and dendritic complexity of the adult brain. Thus, at least five-sixths of dendritic branching occurs postnatally during the period of language development. . . . [M]odern research suggests that enriched experiences may change the neural architecture of the brain long after the initial stages of CNS [central nervous system] development have created the foundation for learning, memory and language development. Changes in synaptic plasticity—the proclivity of synapses and neural circuits to adapt in response to experience—modify changes that, in turn, affect the number and/or the location of synapses (pp. 12–13).

Thus, an ongoing, delayed, or disordered function or element shown in Table 1.1 must be considered in the context of the effects on the child's total developmental framework.

Typical and Atypical Language Development

For a myriad of reasons—some well understood and others as yet unclear—some infants and toddlers fail to move along a developmental course toward attainment of the expected level of communicative competence by their third birthday. Most, if not all, readers of this work have a thorough understanding of typical sequences of language development, probably having completed a specific course in that subject. Several relevant references are provided in Appendix A for readers who would like a quick review of expected sequences of language acquisition during the first 3 years of life.

When children fail to follow the typical course of communicative development, even during the presymbolic period, it is a cause of concern. Approximately 6–10% of infants born each year do not follow the expected developmental course as a result of some disturbance in the synergistic relationships among the basic elements that promote communicative competency. It is estimated that the number of individual infants and toddlers so affected ranges between 630,000 and 1,050,000.[4] For those children and their families, the impact is manifested in social, emotional, behavioral, and preacademic abilities.

Development of communicative competence begins before birth and is pivotal to cognitive, psychoemotional, behavioral, and social development. The ability to comprehend the communication of others (receptive language ability), to process one's emotions and ideas and code the message one wishes to convey (linguistic mapping), and to convey that information to a communicative partner (expressive language ability) is communicative competence. The earliest interactions between mother and infant set the stage for a child's linguistic communicative development. By the end of the first year of life, most babies begin using words meaningfully and rapidly build a repertoire of spoken words and an even larger repertoire of words they understand. During the first years of life, most children master the essentials of oral language: basic phonology, semantics, morphology, syntax, and pragmatics. By 3 years of age, children are usually adept at relating their feelings and experiences in conversing with others.

It is obvious that atypical communicative development can be associated with an array of causal and perpetuating factors, the nature, seriousness, and timing of which affect the prognosis for a favorable outcome. Sometimes the communicative problem is one aspect of a complex of problems that affect the child's health, physical growth, cognitive ability, motor functions, and other areas of development. Sometimes the communicative delay or disorder is the only identified developmental problem.

HISTORICAL PERSPECTIVE OF EARLY INTERVENTION

An understanding of today's approach to early intervention must take into account the parallel efforts of a number of professions and of families of infants, toddlers, and preschool children with special needs. Over the past decade, major advances in knowledge have resulted from contributions of clinicians and researchers in child development and education, medicine and allied health, social services, and other professions. Recent research across a number of professional disciplines, including medicine, nursing, physical therapy, occupational therapy, speech-language pathology, audiology, the biological sciences, social work, and early childhood education, along with clinical experiences of pediatric practitioners, have provided a rich mix of data establishing the value of early intervention for children with developmental delays and disabilities.[16–23]

Education Legislation and Its Role in Development of Early Intervention

Precursors to recent advances in knowledge about working with young children were generated by projects completed in the 1970s and 1980s that generally focused on children in the 3- to 5-year age group, which was then considered the appropriate target for early-intervention efforts. A great deal of what is known about infant-toddler development and effective intervention practices emerged from studies and pilot demonstration programs that followed in the late 1980s and early 1990s. School systems established preschool programs in many states in response to federally funded incentives to serve young children with identified "handicaps." The number of preschool children (ages 3–5 years) served under Part B of IDEA (formerly known as Public Law 94-142) increased from 260,931 in 1986 (under the Education for the Handicapped Act) to 478,617 in 1993 (by which time the reauthorized law was known as *IDEA*).[24] Although results of the early model programs and the subsequent proliferation of preschool programs for children with special needs were giant steps forward, groundwork laid during that time period clearly indicated that habilitation for young children with developmental delays and disabilities needed to be undertaken much earlier than the preschool years to be optimally effective.

From the beginning, states were given the option under Public Law 94-142 (Education for the Handicapped Act) to establish programs for children from birth to 21 years of age. States were mandated to serve children from 6 to 21 years of age and encouraged to serve preschool children in the 3- to 5-year age group. In 1990, the Education for the Handicapped Act was reauthorized by Congress under a different title (IDEA).[25] In 1986, an amendment to the act was added in the form of Public Law 99-457,[26] which was later amended as Public Law 102-119 and became known as *Part H*.[27]

Part H mandated that participating states that had not already done so establish programs for 3- to 5-year-old children with special needs. Further, it encouraged states, using self-determined guidelines, to establish a multidisciplinary, community-based, family-focused, interagency system of services for infants and toddlers with special needs and their families. The unique features of Part H included (1) a 5-year planning period during which funding was provided to participating states to get their system up and running; (2) the authority of each state to name its own Lead Agency to oversee establishment and administration of the system; (3) the authority of each state to establish its own eligibility requirements for participation in the system, so long as children with medical diagnoses indicative of developmental delays or disabilities and those with established delays or disparities were included; (4) a requirement that the needs of *families* of eligible children be addressed to assist them in enhancing their child's optimal development; (5) the authority of each state to develop its own procedures and guidelines to see that an Individual Family Service Plan is in place for each family with an eligible child; (6) unprecedented short timelines to comply with required assessment and evaluation processes to establish eligibility for services following referral of a child; (7) a mandate of family service coordination (previously referred to as *case management*); and (8) the provision of services, to the extent possible, in naturalistic environments. *Naturalistic environments* were defined as those in which children of the same age who do not have developmental disabilities would normally be found; this is generally interpreted as homes and child care facilities.

The intent of Part H legislation was clearly to promote optimal development of infants and toddlers with special needs. In many states, especially in those whose Lead Agency is the state department of education, the focus on preparing children for school experiences has become a primary focus of Part H efforts. In fact, many children who transition out of the Part H system are transitioned to Part B (special education) programs for preschool children with special needs.

Reauthorization of IDEA in 1997 changed the infant-toddler statutory reference from Part H to Part C, strengthened the role of families, and expanded the requirements for transition planning.[11]

From the perspective of policy makers and legislators who allocate and administer taxpayer dollars, it is important to see that children are prepared to enter school ready to learn (a theme articulated in those very words in the Goals 2000 education initiative). Interestingly, that effort to date has not taken particular notice of that preparation's dependence on communicative competence, despite the fact that most children in "noncategorical preschool" programs (which succeeded "preschool programs for the handicapped") have significant delays in communication skills.

Communicative Competence and Education

From the perspective of performance in the classroom, communicative competence is *the basic academic skill*—a fact that is so fundamental that it is often overlooked. Young children with communicative disorders have no capacity for personal comparison of their language systems with those of their peers. There is generally no physical pain or discomfort associated with communicative delays or impairments; they do not portend physical degeneration or other "scientifically measurable" deficiencies; they are not fatal; and they are usually not accompanied by traits that distinguish affected children from their age peers. Often, children with communicative difficulties are judged by parents, teachers, or other adults to be "immature" or "slow." It is usually not until the child is expected to be able to transfer oral-communication skills to deriving meaning from new sets of symbols (i.e., letters and numerals) in literacy tasks that the language difficulty becomes evident. The very complexity of the processes involved—and their interdependency—seem too often to mitigate against actions that can be taken early on to address difficulties in communicative development, especially in the absence of accompanying physical impairments.[28] Since the passage of Part H, all states have elected to participate, and many families and children from birth to 36 months of age are being served in early-intervention programs.

Preparation for literacy, however important, cannot be the total focus of the impact of delays and disorders of communicative development; the entirety of a child's life is affected when significant communication difficulties are present.

Health Care and Early Intervention

Advances in providing prenatal care in typical and high-risk pregnancies, dramatic improvements in neonatology, and the availability of increasingly effective pharmacologic management for a variety of diseases have contributed to the medical community's ability to preserve the lives of infants who in earlier times would not have survived. It is not uncommon today for babies born at 6 months gestation to survive. Only a few years ago, children born with birth weights of less than 1,500 g were not considered viable; now infants born at 1,000 g (and sometimes less) are surviving, thanks to advances in knowledge and technology.

Advances in neonatal care extend beyond the availability of specialized equipment, pharmacologic products, and highly trained medical practitioners. Developmental specialists in nursing, occupational therapy, physical therapy, and medical social work contribute to improved outcomes for compromised babies and their families. The work of Heidelese Als and her colleagues has changed the concept of the nurturing environment of the NICU.[29-35] When the best practices are used, lights are dimmed and noise levels are lowered to reduce the sensory stimulation with which the fragile newborns have to contend. In some units, family members and volunteer staff offer skin-to-skin contact ("kangaroo care") for babies who were born too soon. The emotional needs of the infants and their families are being given high priority in implementing treatment that previously focused only on the medical requirements called for simply to preserve life. Procedures to enhance the infant's quality of life, attachment, and emotional adjustment are considered important parts of the treatment plans for at-risk babies.

It has become relatively commonplace for SLPs in large hospitals to be included as members of the NICU team. In such cases, SLPs participate in developmental assessment; counsel families and professional colleagues in early communicative interactions between infants and their caregivers; and assist physicians, nursing staff, and occupational therapists in determining whether a given infant is ready for oral feedings and how that process can be optimized by use of specialized feeding equipment and appropriate positioning. These roles for the SLP are relatively new and obviously require specialized training and skills. More detailed information about the role of the SLP in the NICU is covered in Chapter 5.

Audiologists also play an important role in newborn care. Electrophysiologic measurements of integrity of the auditory system, along with traditional audiometric assessment, have become commonplace in dealing with the needs of infants and toddlers. Early detection of hearing impairment and early application of appropriate habilitation strategies—including early fitting of amplification when indicated—have contributed to improved developmental outcomes for hearing-impaired children. Additional information about assessment and management for hearing impairment in infants and toddlers is provided in Chapters 6 and 9.

The results of advances in prenatal and neonatal care are mixed. On one hand, ever-increasing numbers of infants are surviving preterm delivery; many medically compromised infants are being treated successfully; and early management of some congenital anomalies is making it possible for larger numbers of children to look forward to brighter futures. On the other hand, it is impossible to establish conditions that guarantee a "normal" developmental course for all of these infants. Many survivors continue to have problems that compromise their development in one or more areas. Some of the residual impairments are highly visible (as in cerebral palsy, severe craniofacial anomalies, and some syndromes), while others are not superficially apparent (as in certain chronic diseases, some neurologic conditions, most receptive communicative disorders, and some expressive communicative disorders). The bottom line is that there are larger numbers of children surviving with conditions that are likely to be predictive of significant developmental delays or disorders, which require management by practitioners from many professional disciplines.

Physicians who care for infants and toddlers have children other than NICU "graduates" among their patients. The majority of infants are not admitted to NICUs; most children born in U.S. hospitals are admitted for a day or two to regular newborn nurseries or are allowed to room-in with their mothers during a brief hospital confinement. Additionally, home births attended by midwives or nurse practitioners are prevalent in some parts of the country. Infants and toddlers who appear to be physically healthy sometimes exhibit significant developmental delays or disorders that may or may not be detected by their physicians. The time pressures imposed by busy medical practices combined with scant training in medical schools related to identification and management of nondisease-related delays and disorders of early childhood often result in inappropriate attention to those problems and help to explain why so many children are reaching the age of school entry before the seriousness of the problems is revealed.

The American Academy of Pediatrics (AAP) and various public health agencies, including the National Institutes of Health, have made significant efforts to address these issues. Reduction of infant mortality rates has been a common goal of all groups, as has improving child (and maternal) health. Public awareness campaigns promoting early and continuous prenatal care; the federally funded nutrition program for women, infants, and children, the establishment of Kid-Med centers to provide community-based well-child health care; and the Medical Home initiative of the AAP are all examples of nationwide efforts to improve health care for children from conception on.

Unfortunately, the country is battling other societal problems that mitigate against the efforts of those promoting child health and welfare. The explosion of drug use among those in their child-bearing years, the spread of autoimmune deficiency diseases (e.g., acquired immunodeficiency syndrome), the renewed incidence of sexually transmitted diseases (including syphilis), the increased numbers of smokers among teens and young adults, and the widespread abuse of alcohol in that age group are of concern because of potential increases in developmental disabilities among infants and toddlers born to affected mothers. The combination of low socioeconomic status and low educational attainment of mothers is a further problem that places infants and toddlers at risk for developmental delays and disabilities.[36] Neither the medical community alone nor in conjunction with members of the educational community can hope to deal with problems of this magnitude. Solutions—if they are to be found—must involve political, legal, medical, educational, religious, family, and individual efforts.

FAMILIES, BABIES, AND EARLY INTERVENTION

Through the years, families of children with atypical developmental patterns have struggled to find ways to help their children. In this country, attitudes toward families of children with special needs have undergone significant changes. Child protection laws, education legislation that mandates services to families of infants and toddlers with special needs, development of standards of practices among medical and allied health professions dealing with the youngest pediatric populations, public health legislation, and other developments of recent times are all reflective of society's attempts to address the issues with which every family with a special-needs child deals.

From an individual family's perspective, however knowledgeable they are about the availability or scarcity of public policies to cover their particular situation, issues related to their child's development, including communication development, are more personal. The issues involve relationships between the child and other members of the family. Parents face any problem involving their child's development with a set of issues unique to their own experiences. Their emotions, expectations, perceptions, levels of information and abilities to process it, present concerns, priorities, and coping mechanisms are factors that affect their decision making. These factors also affect the family's ongoing relationships with professionals who are in the picture *because* of the child's atypical development and perhaps only for that reason. All families balance a plethora of day-to-day demands on their time, energy, attention, and resources. A family with a child whose developmental problems require the attention of a number of professionals, which is typical of many families who are referred to communicative disorders specialists, may experience a significant amount of stress as they parcel out their time, energy, and other resources to meet the needs of their young child. Figure 1.1 illustrates the demands that face many such families. Each of the elements depicted has positive and negative aspects, as the family attempts to balance daily activities and simultaneously attend to the needs of their atypically developing child.

Any consideration of the perspectives of families must take into account the fact that very few families *expect* to be dealing with anything but a healthy, typically developing child. Consider the implications and functional impact on emotional, financial, marital, and social aspects of family functioning of the birth of a child whose problems require immediate and difficult decisions on the part of the parents with respect to medical or surgical treatment options, impose unexpected and huge financial hardships related to extended stays in NICUs, or result in the need for long-term management of congenital or acquired conditions or diseases. It takes time to adjust to what life is like, when compared with what the parents expected life to be like as they anticipated the birth of a healthy child. Alternatively, if the child appeared to be healthy at birth and experienced no major medical problems, consider the impact of a gradual discovery that the child's development is not proceeding along a typical path.

The growing anxieties—or dealing with the unanticipated pronouncement by a professional whose assessment has revealed a "deficit" or "significant delay"—of whether the child will be able to deal with social situations, adjust to a child care setting, and succeed in school when the time comes are difficult for

Figure 1.1 Child and family.

the family. Some families are better able than others to cope, to identify and use available resources to promote their child's development, and to advocate for their child. It is part of the professional's role to assist those families who need support in those endeavors and promote their innate ability to make choices that meet their own and their child's needs. Early interventionists refer to that goal as *empowering* the family. Families often comment that they are already "empowered" to make such decisions; what they need is access to the information that enables them to make informed decisions that assist them in optimizing their child's development.

Communication Disorders Specialists and Early Intervention

The frame of reference for understanding the impact of atypical communicative development must include knowledge that the majority of children receiving special education services in the schools, regardless of their primary diagnosis or "eligibility label," receive speech-language therapy services. Obviously, these children did not suddenly develop communication delays or disorders at the time of school entry. The fact that they have a communication delay or disorder at the time they enter school places them at risk for academic difficulties in reading and other literacy-based subjects, *because literacy skills are built on the foundation of oral-language competencies.*[28,37] Research indicates that a substantial number of children with many special-education service eligibility labels have coexisting communication delays, disorders, or both. The most heavily documented problems in which communication development is also affected are autism, attention-deficit hyperactivity disorder, cerebral palsy, and certain genetic syndromes. In fact, the presence of a communication disorder or significant delay is a hallmark for the diagnosis itself in many instances. This issue is addressed more specifically in Chapters 2 and 7.

Until recently, early communication delays were generally not thought of as being especially noteworthy by the medical community. Parents who exhibited concern about their child's late talking were frequently told by their pediatricians that a referral would be made only if the problem persisted past the age of 3. Information emerging from infant research on cognitive, social, emotional, sensory, and physical factors that contribute to the development of speech and language long before the emergence of the spoken word has become more readily available with advances in, and widespread use of, information technology. Access to the research knowledge base combined with recognition of the advantages of early intervention and efforts of the AAP to encourage physician referrals to early intervention services are changing the way in which the medical community deals with high-incidence, low-visibility problems in the pediatric population. The availability of a legitimate medical diagnostic code for "developmental delay" has also contributed to the emergence of attention to developmental problems earlier in the child's life.[7]

Years before the age of school entry (and introduction to literacy), children with communicative difficulties are at risk for a variety of other problems. Children who have problems communicating are at risk for atypical social development. Early interactions with significant others are adversely affected when the child is not typically responsive to the efforts of caregivers. Research indicates that children with impaired early interactive and preintentional communicative abilities are responded to differently by their parents and other caregivers.[38–40] Specific preintentional communication intervention strategies are indicated when this is the case. SLPs can be called on to train caregivers to look for small changes in the child's responses to their bids for interaction, rather than simply noting the absence of the expected behaviors of typically developing infants. Behaviors of toddlers who are frustrated by an inadequate ability to convey their feelings through language are often problematic, compounding the frustrations of their families and other caregivers who wish they could interpret what the child is trying to convey but often cannot. The problematic behavior (e.g., withdrawal, excessive dependence, frequent tantrums) in turn often generates a set of issues that sometimes become the primary focus of the family or daycare provider, who often do not consider the communicative difficulty as a precipitator of the behavioral problem.[16] Speech-language specialists can serve as consultants to families and daycare providers to help deal with such situations, helping the adults deal effectively with behavior modification when communicative impairment is the underlying factor triggering undesirable behaviors.

Some conditions associated with communicative delays and disorders have an adverse effect on the child's physical development. Feeding and swallowing difficulties can be present in the child with tongue mobility difficulties or palatal anomalies observed by the SLP. The infant with a persistent odd quality of cry may be referred by the SLP to an otorhinolaryngologist (i.e., ear, nose, and throat specialist) for evaluation of specific physical problems (e.g., choanal atresia, laryngeal polypoid growths, vocal fold paresis or unilateral paralysis, submucous or overt palatal cleft). Over time, these specific physical problems could underlie compensatory motor adjustments that impact growth patterns of bony- or soft-tissue structures or interfere with adequate nutrition. Toddlers with extremely poor articulation abilities may have ankylosis of the lingual frenum with resultant physical growth deformities of dental or mandibular structures. These issues are dealt with in more detail in Chapter 7.

High-Incidence, Low-Visibility Disorders

Children with delays and disorders affecting communication development comprise a large portion of the high-incidence, low-visibility population. While there is a segment of the pediatric population with high-visibility, low-incidence developmental disabilities associated with atypical communicative development (e.g., craniofacial anomalies, syndromes with characteristic physical features such as Down syndrome), the majority of children with delayed or disordered communicative development look like other children in their age groups. It is often *because* they "look normal" that their difficulties with communicative development are downplayed or overlooked entirely. It takes continuing efforts on the part of those who understand the impact of communicative impairments to educate the public and the professional community to the pervasiveness of the problem and its potential to adversely affect other areas of development. Demonstration through clinical programs that early intervention for communication problems can be effective must be coupled with ongoing communication with other professionals who work with the population and with families. Part of the professional role of the communicative-disorders specialist serving this population must be to undertake these responsibilities.[41]

MANAGED CARE AND EARLY INTERVENTION

The health care environment, including that segment relating to early intervention, is demanding adjustment to the rapid proliferation of managed care plans that have arisen in response to mushrooming health care costs. Under managed care plans, primary care providers (PCPs) (i.e., licensed obstetricians, pediatricians, and family practitioners) control access to other services: In effect, they are the gatekeepers for all health services. Members of a managed care plan are required to access services through the PCP. A feature of many, if not most, managed care plans is capitation. *Capitation* is a basic fee paid to participating PCPs for each member of the plan based on a formula devised by the managed care plan administrators or negotiated between the contracted PCPs and plan administrators. The PCP is awarded a fixed dollar amount under the contractual arrangement. That dollar amount is designed to cover charges for all care provided to plan members during a specified term. If the PCP manages to "save" costs by reducing referral to specialists and subspecialists and limiting expensive testing procedures, hospital admissions, or both, any dollars remaining in the fund at the end of a fixed time period specified in the contract are awarded to the PCP as a reward for conserving resources. Capitation practices are a subject of great debate with respect to ethical decision making, the care that is in the best interests of patient-health outcomes, and the roles of specialists and subspecialists in medicine and allied health fields (e.g., speech-language pathology, occupational therapy, physical therapy, audiology).[42]

Obviously the PCP's role as gatekeeper, or referring agent, has taken on overtones of personal economics that are different from the issues involved before the advent of managed care. Will the hard-won knowledge that a child with developmental delays or disabilities can profit from intervention before the age of 3 years be ignored by persons with authority to make referrals in the interest of protecting the capitation limit? The full impact of managed care plans has yet to be realized, and, in time, there will undoubtedly be changes in the operations of some plans. Practitioners who rely on the PCP for referrals must monitor this situation carefully, if they hope to survive in this environment. An example of the issue for communicative disorders specialists is found in the denial of payment for language-therapy services rendered to a child of a managed care plan participant because the PCP did not make the referral for that service. Precertification for services is a common requirement of managed care plans. Precertification requires PCP referral. It is awarded normally for a specified number of visits, with authority to extend the treatment for additional visits dependent on documentation satisfactory to the managed care certification officer (who may or may not be knowledgeable about communication-therapy regimes) that the extension is warranted. This is a critical issue for practitioners who are required by Public Law 102-119 and recent amendments to IDEA (Public Law 205-17, Part C, which pertains to the population from birth to 3 years of age) to serve infants and toddlers in naturalistic environments to the extent possible. This is problematic because homes and child care centers do not qualify as health care centers, and many early-intervention programs are operated through community organizations (e.g., the Association for Retarded Citizens) or as a service of local schools. One bright spot is that at least one health maintenance organization has carved out a special division to handle infants and toddlers with special needs.[43]

Maintaining ongoing lines of communication with PCPs is a crucial issue.[44,45] Assisting them in understanding why early referrals are critical is essential. Dealing with the certification officer at the administrative offices of managed care plans is a new area in which professional skills are needed. Understanding what a particular plan requires by way of authorization for services is a particular challenge, because plans differ in their requirements.

FRAMEWORK OF THE FAMILY AND PROFESSIONAL TEAM

An immediate realization of professionals who work with the infant-toddler population is that their families are the true decision makers with respect to the care the children receive. Professionals can and do make recommendations about appropriate management options, suggest intervention or treatment strategies, and provide pertinent information; ultimately, however, the family chooses the paths to take or whether to select any path at all. Whether the family is forced to deal with difficult decisions at the time their child is born (e.g., authorizing surgery or special treatment, selecting one medical specialist over another, finding a way to pay for expensive care for their child with a congenital condition) or faces a set of different decisions later, either as a result of a traumatic event that leaves the child with a disability or through realization that the child's developmental course is impaired, a great deal of emotional energy and personal tension can be expected. Families move through adjustments at varying rates and with varying degrees of comfort and success. Adjustment is not the same for all members of the family, nor are the issues involved given equal weight by all members of the family. Coping mechanisms vary within the family. Coping and adjustment to a child's developmental delays or disorders is not linear: There are sometimes slow steps forward, and occasionally there are leaps forward only to be followed by a return to an earlier level of dealing with the situation. There can be short or long periods of "plateau," when the family chooses not to deal with the issues or cannot do so for some reason.

The concerns, priorities, and resources of the family may be different from those of the professionals. When there is intersection of family and professional goals to promote the best outcome for the child, opportunities for effective teaming between families and professionals are created.

The author's experiences with families mirrors what is found in the research literature with respect to coping and adjustment. Some families (or members of families) are open and responsive, seek information, and quickly follow through on suggestions and management strategies, while others appear to be resistant to any suggestion that something should or could be done, even to the point of denying (overtly or covertly) that a problem exists. Still others wax and wane in their involvement with intervention or treatment plans, even if they helped to create them. Such responses can be attributed to human nature and are not necessarily a comment on either the character traits of family members or the skills of the professionals involved. Additionally, families sometimes report that they cannot work with certain professionals because of their inflexibility or insistence on following a particular course of treatment or management that is unacceptable to the family. The family's choices may be based on religious beliefs, child-rearing practices, social or cultural values, or simply intuition. With the exceptions of parental choices that result in criminal or medical neglect or child abuse, parents are free to make those choices that make the most sense for their families.

As professionals, we must keep reminding ourselves that families are dealing with a myriad of difficult decisions, including but not limited to those we have placed before them. Their lives are more complex than the slices of it with which we are involved because of a particular child. They move at their own pace. Our responsibility is to provide them with enough information to make those decisions that make the most sense to them. We must be open to listening to what their concerns and priorities are. We must also find out what their supports and resources are.

Although the timing of communication intervention is critical and sometimes crucial to a desired outcome, families may not see the situation through the same lens that we use. The family is dealing with balancing the costs of some services against other financial priorities in their lives. Families who are engaged with multiple members of the early-intervention professional team (who can but probably do not practice in the same setting) also have to balance appointment schedules, transportation arrangements, and other matters, in addition to caring for the child and the needs of other family members. Demands of the managed care system, program-eligibility requirements, lifetime insurance caps, availability of and accessibility to services, medications, and needed equipment can take precedence over a professional's desire for an immediate decision by the family about a management recommendation.

Another matter requiring the attention of the family and practitioners with whom they work is the extent to which family members, particularly the mother or primary caregiver, desire to function as members of the early-intervention team. For many people, this concept is not readily acceptable. Their cultural background, values, prior life experiences, educational background, socioeconomic status, belief system, and expectations (especially about disabilities and relationships with professionals) all bear on their concept of what it means to be a team member. Although many professionals have adopted the stance that team membership is the ideal way of addressing early-intervention activities, we must keep in mind that in most cases the whole experience of early intervention is new to every family with whom we come in contact.

Establishing a satisfactory working relationship with any family takes time and patience on the part of both the professional and family members as they adjust to each other and define both their commitment to the process and their expectations of one another. The professional must be able to provide the information and tools with which the family can operate as true partners, if they choose to do so.

SERVICE-DELIVERY MODELS IN EARLY INTERVENTION

Infants and toddlers who have or are at risk for communicative disorders may come to the attention of the SLP through referrals to developmental programs or through clinical programs. Developmental programs are often conducted under the auspices of community-based agencies and operate in keeping with the mandates of Part H/Part C of IDEA. Clinical programs more traditionally operate in health care settings and private practices. They tend to be "center based"—that is, families take their children to the professional. Conversely, Part H/Part C mandate that services be delivered, to the extent possible, in naturalistic environments, which requires professionals to travel.[46] Center-based programs are not prohibited by Part H/Part C legislation, but very young children do not typically attend habilitative programs. The very young child's normal environment is the home, and many regularly attend child care during their parents' working hours. Increasingly, the philosophies of both developmental programs and clinical programs are being applied in meeting the needs of atypically developing young children and their families when communicative problems are the primary issue. Developmentally appropriate practices are the hallmark against which every management program should be measured.

Under IDEA *families* are also eligible for services if their children qualify.[46] Many children who could profit from early intervention do not qualify for Part H/Part C services, however, either because their developmental delays are "not serious enough" to meet their state's eligibility criteria, or because the nature of the risk is excluded from defined eligibility guidelines. For example, environmentally at-risk children (especially those whose low family socioeconomic status is combined with the mother's low educational achievement level) constitute a group who could profit from early intervention.[47] Although states are encouraged to include at-risk groups in their eligibility criteria, financial considerations are substantial, and children in environmentally at-risk groups are omitted from eligibility definitions in most states.

Eligibility for services under clinical service delivery models varies considerably across agencies and practices. As with the Part H/Part C model, it is most likely that children who are referred early in life for SLP services under the clinical model are infants or toddlers with physical anomalies (especially craniofacial anomalies), hearing impairment, and those who are multiply handicapped. Eligibility, especially in the private sector, is often dictated by family income level or insurance coverage or other factors unrelated to the child's developmental needs. It should be noted that some families take longer than others to adjust to the many facets of the child's condition and to changes in their own lives that can ensue. Developmental habilitation awaits their readiness to seek it. When they do seek such services, they may choose to start with only one service, adding others as they feel or recognize the need to do so. It is particularly important that all professionals on the child's habilitative team appreciate the advantages of approaching development from the perspective of parallel developmental maturation, of taking advantage of synaptogenesis during the early years of life, and of involving a collaborative team effort to achieve optimal outcomes for affected children and their families.

WHAT ABOUT THE FAMILY: ARE THE CHOICES ONLY EITHER-OR?

As SLPs attempt to forge effective parent-professional partnerships, they must acknowledge that just as individuals differ, families are different. The definition of family has changed from the idea of being exclusively comprised of two parents, one or more children, and extended family (i.e., grandparents, aunts, uncles, and cousins). Large numbers of children grow up in single-parent households, often headed by women. Close friends or intimates not related by blood are sometimes considered members of the family and function as such, regardless of whether they live under the same roof. Adoptive or foster families may be responsible for the child. Blood-related extended family members do not live under the same roof in most families, as was once a common practice, although this practice varies considerably across cultural groups. In homes where there are two parents, both may work outside the home, leaving the child during most waking hours in the hands of child care providers in home-based or center-based programs. Staff members of such centers can change often, introducing the child to new faces on a fairly frequent basis. Identification with a "primary caregiver" can be tenuous with some children. These issues are addressed in more detail in Chapter 7, as they can affect child development and planning and implementing management of communicative difficulties. Ultimately, decisions regarding the child still rest in the hands of the parent(s), of course, but factors influencing the decision-making process must be considered by professionals who work with the child and family.

Open-minded professionals recognize that it is possible to combine the service delivery models discussed above to the advantage of all concerned. Children and their families may qualify for Part H/Part C services at some points in time and not at others. Families may prefer to use services of a private practitioner or of a particular clinical program at certain points in the child's life or may choose to address specific needs they feel may be more appropriately handled by a particular practitioner who is not part of the IDEA system. At other times, families may wish to take advantage of the multidisciplinary approach offered through the Part H/Part C service model or some specialized pediatric clinical practices. Thus, the professional finds that the family's choice of options can vary over time, according to their perception of the child's needs, their priorities, and their resources.

Challenges that may be new to professionals are understanding the scope of available options, sharing information with the family so that they can understand the bases of professional recommendations, communicating openly with the family about advantages and disadvantages of various service-delivery systems, and supporting the family in their choice of services for their child and themselves. Table 1.2 provides an overview of the basic service-delivery models that provide the framework for services to infants and toddlers with or at high risk for disabilities and their families.

PROFESSIONAL COMPETENCIES

Under whatever service-delivery model employed (the parents may or may not know what model is being applied by a given practice or agency), it is imperative that practitioners who work with infants and toddlers with or at risk for developmental disabilities possess the essential competencies, knowledge base, and experiential background. The American Speech-Language-Hearing Association published guidelines for professionals who work with infants and toddlers.[48] Additionally, certain competencies are outlined in Part H/Part C implementation rules and regulations. Multidisciplinary guidelines have been developed by the Division of Early Childhood of the Council for Exceptional Children.[49] Suggested guidelines for physicians dealing with developmentally disabled children have been published by the AAP.[50] Copies of the guidelines are available from those organizations.

Families who entrust their children to professionals, often at times of emotional and financial stress, anticipate that they will deal with practitioners who can guide them appropriately as they face making decisions that have the potential to alter their children's lives. Regardless of socioeconomic status, level of intelligence, educational background, or family composition, parents are anxious to secure the best available treatment for their children's needs. Some may have an unrealistic expectation about a possible "cure" for serious disabilities with no known remedy; over time, the family's expectations will become more realistic as a result of their interactions with professionals and through their own life experiences. Professionals must strike a critical balance between the family's hopes for the future of each child and appropriate management leading to optimal developmental outcomes for each child.

The following chapters of this work focus on specific issues of diagnosis, assessment, and management for communication disorders.

Table 1.2 Comparative Features of Various Service Delivery Models

Model	Likely Service Setting	Population Served and Approaches Used	Focus
Clinical	Hospital or other medical setting (e.g., NICU) Out-patient services Health care centers, practices, or programs Specialized multidisciplinary teams (e.g., craniofacial anomalies teams, cleft lip or cleft palate teams, feeding teams)	Newborns, infants, and toddlers are served. The service is child centered. The service relies heavily on professional expertise for guidance and selection of treatment and care options. The service includes a well-established chain of command (lines of authority). Parents rely heavily on professionals' knowledge and expertise. Parents are given options regarding choices, receive training in specialized procedures, and are provided information regarding community resources.	Prevention Diagnosis Assessment Discharge planning Team collaboration Parent training and education Health, wellness, and promotion of development
Clinical	Solo or group SLP practice, such as traditional center-based private practice with or without off-site consultants	The population can be limited to or only service portions of the birth to 3-year-old population, depending on structure of the clinical practice. The SLP or audiologist may contract with various agencies to provide services at other than office sites.	Unidisciplinary, child-centered therapy Family participation directed by practitioner in keeping with clinical goals
Group or multidisciplinary	Professional practice, often office-group practice with or without off-site consultants	Population served varies from inclusion of birth to 3-year-old children and their families to inclusion of selected subgroups (e.g., autism, cerebral palsy, language disorders). Services are dictated by the composition of target group(s).	Child-centered Dependent to a large extent on combination of disciplines comprising the team, (e.g., physical therapy, occupational therapy, and SLP; psychology and educa-

Model	Likely Service Setting	Population Served and Approaches Used	Focus
		Services are often specific to needs of children with developmental or physical health needs or those with designated conditions or diagnoses.	tion; medicine, social work, SLP, and psychology)
Developmental	Multidisciplinary early intervention teams (which can be center based or combination home based and center based)	Ages served vary from comprehensive inclusion of birth to 3-year-old children and their families to selected groups (e.g., mental retardation, cerebral palsy, autism). Services are usually family focused and governed by federal and state early intervention statutes. Management by IFSP is commonly used, whether or not it is required by law. Services are based on family priorities, and objectives are related to enhancing the child's development.	Services fall between clinical and educational models Historic origins often traced to developmental disability programs, parent-funded centers for specific problems, or to university training or research programs
Developmental	Multidisciplinary developmental assessment teams that can operate in conjunction with the following: Health care centers Hospital units Developmental disability centers Local education agencies Centers sponsored by civic organizations (e.g., SERTOMA, Scottish Rite, Easter Seal Society)	The population served can include all of the birth to 3-year-old population and their families or be limited by policy or statutory regulation to a segment thereof. Programs offer specialized assessment leading to referral elsewhere for treatment, therapy, or intervention.	Diagnosis and assessment for designated purposes conducted in highly specialized settings Generally child-centered, but can be more family focused

NICU = neonatal intensive care unit; SLP = speech-language pathology/ist; IFSP = individual family service plan.

REFERENCES

1. Office of the Assistant Secretary for Planning and Evaluation, U.S. Department of Health and Human Services. ASPE Research Notes. January 1995.
2. U.S. Department of Education. Seventeenth Report to Congress on the Implementation of Individuals with Disabilities Education Act. 1995.
3. Newacheck PW, Taylor WR. Childhood chronic illness: prevalence, severity, and impact. Am J Public Health 1992;82:364.
4. Wenger BL, Kaye HS, LaPlante MP. Disabilities Among Children. Disability Statistics Abstract, no. 15. Washington, DC: U.S. Department of Education, National Institute on NIDRR Outcome, 1996.
5. U.S. Department of Health and Human Services/Public Health Service. Disabilities among children age ≤17 years—United States, 1991–1992. MMWR Morb Mortal Wkly Rep 1995;44:33.
6. American Medical Association. Physicians' Current Procedural Terminology. Chicago: CPT Intellectual Property Services, American Medical Association, 1996.
7. American Medical Association. International Classification of Diseases (9th ed). Clinical Modification. Dover, DE: American Medical Association, 1996.
8. American Academy of Pediatrics. The Classification of Child and Adolescent Mental Diagnoses in Primary Care: Diagnostic and Statistical Manual for Primary Care (DSM-PC) Child and Adolescent Version. Elk Grove Village, IL: AAP Division of Publications, 1997.
9. American Psychiatric Association. Diagnostic and Statistical Manual of Mental Disorders (4th ed). Washington, DC: American Psychological Association, 1996.
10. Zero to Three/National Center for Clinical Infant Programs. Diagnostic Classification: 0–3—Diagnostic Classification of Mental Health and Developmental Disorders of Infancy and Early Childhood. Arlington, VA: Zero to Three/National Center for Clinical Infant Programs, 1994.
11. Individuals with Disabilities Education Act Amendments of 1991. Pub L No. 102-119.
12. Rehabilitation Act of 1973. Sec. 504 (34 CFR 104.3 [j]).
13. OSEP's Hehir voices concern about need for more child-find in Part H. Early Child Rep 1996;7:7.
14. Fewell R. Educator says research points to need for more aid for children with less severe disabilities [excerpts from keynote address of Rebecca Fewell at the 1996 conference of the Division of Early Childhood]. Early Child Rep 1997;8:3.
15. Hallett T, Proctor A. Maturation of the central nervous system as related to communication and cognitive development. Infants Young Child 1986;8:1.
16. Prizant BM, Meyer EC. Socioemotional aspects of language and social-communication disorders in young children. Am J Speech-Lang Pathol 1993;2:56.
17. Catts HW. The relationship between speech-language impairments and reading disabilities. J Speech Hear Res 1993;36:948.
18. Lockwood SL. Early speech and language indicators for later learning problems: recognizing a language organization disorder. Infants Young Child 1994;7:43.
19. Menyuk P. Syntactic and Reading Disabilities. In J Stark, P Menyuk, S Wurtzel (eds), Language Learning and Reading Disabilities: A New Decade. New York: Queens College Press, 1980.
20. Ramey CT, Bryan DM, Wasik BH, et al. Infant health and development program for low birth weight premature infants: program elements, family participation, and child intelligence. Pediatrics 1992;89:454.
21. Bryant DM, Ramey CT. An Analysis of the Effectiveness of Early Intervention Programs for Environmentally At-Risk Children. In M Guralnick, FC Bennett (eds), Effectiveness of Early Intervention. Orlando, FL: Academic Press, 1987;33.

22. Campbell RA, Ramey CT. Effects of early intervention on intellectual and academic achievement: a follow-up study of children from low-income families. Child Dev 1994;65:684.
23. Shonkoff JP, Hauser-Cram P. Early intervention for disabled infants and their families: a quantitative analysis. Pediatrics 1987;80:650.
24. Preschool program data. Early Child Rep 1994;5:7.
25. Education for the Handicapped Act of 1975. Pub L No. 94-142.
26. Amendments to the Education for the Handicapped Act of 1986. Pub L No. 99-457.
27. Individuals with Disabilities Education Act of 1990. Pub L No. 101-476.
28. Wetherby AM, Prizant BM. Toward Earlier Identification of Communication and Language Problems in Young Children. In SJ Meisels, E Fenichel (eds), New Visions for the Developmental Assessment of Infants and Young Children. Washington, DC: Zero to Three/National Center for Clinical Infant Programs, 1996;289.
29. Alfonso DD, Wahlberg V, Persson B. Exploration of mothers' reactions to the kangaroo method of prematurity care. Neonatal Network 1989;7:43.
30. Als H. Individualized, Family-Focused Developmental Care for the Very Low Birthweight Preterm Infant in the NICU. In SL Friedman, MD Sigman (eds), Advances in Applied Developmental Psychology (Vol. 6). Norwood, NJ: Ablex, 1992;341.
31. Becker PT, Grunwald PC, Moorman J, Stuhr S. Outcomes of developmentally supportive nursing care for very low birthweight infants. Nurs Res 1991;40:150.
32. Lawhon G, Melzar A. Developmentally Supportive Interventions. In JP Cloherty, AR Stark (eds), Manual of Neonatal Care (3rd ed). Boston: Little, Brown, 1991;581.
33. McCormick MC. Advances in Neonatal Intensive Care Technology and Their Possible Impact on the Development of Low Birthweight Infants. In SL Friedman, MD Sigman (eds), The Psychological Development of Low-Birthweight Children: Advances in Applied Developmental Psychology. Norwood, NJ: Ablex, 1992;37.
34. Parker SJ, Zahr LK, Cole JG, Brecht M. Outcome after developmental intervention in the neonatal intensive care unit for mothers of preterm infants with low socioeconomic status. J Pediatr 1992;120:780.
35. Schmidt E, Wittreich G. Care of the Abnormal Newborn: A Random Controlled Clinical Trial Study of the "Kangaroo Method of Care for the Low Birth-Weight Newborns." Paper presented at the 1996 World Health Organization Interregional Conference on Appropriate Technology Following Birth, Rome, Italy.
36. Bendersky M, Lewis M. Environmental risk, biological risk, and developmental outcome. Dev Psychol 1994;30:484.
37. Scarborough HS. Very early language deficits in dyslexic children. Child Dev 1990;61:1728.
38. Barnard KE, Kelly JF. Assessment of Parent-Child Interaction. In SJ Meisels, JP Shonkoff (eds), Handbook of Early Childhood Intervention. Cambridge, MA: Cambridge University Press, 1990;278.
39. Barnard KE. Influencing Parent-Child Interactions for Children at Risk. In M Guralnick (ed), The Effectiveness of Early Intervention. Baltimore: Paul H. Brookes, 1997;249.
40. Hudson KM, Giardino AP. Child Abuse and Neglect. In SJ Meisels, JP Shonkoff (eds), Handbook of Early Childhood Intervention. Cambridge, MA: Cambridge University Press, 1997;278.
41. Stark RE. Early language intervention: when, why, how? Infants Young Child 1989;1:44.
42. Shapland C. Be aware that managed care can affect children with disabilities. Pacesetter 1997;20:12.
43. HMO makes an important connection to early intervention. Early Child Rep 1996;7:1.
44. Droter D. But where are the data? Planning services for infants and families in an era of managed care. Infants Young Child 1996;9:vi.

45. Barnett WS, Escobar CM. Economic Costs and Benefits of Early Intervention. In S Meisels, JP Shonkoff (eds), Handbook of Early Childhood Intervention. Cambridge, MA: Cambridge University Press, 1990;560.
46. U.S. Department of Education. Early intervention program for infants and toddlers with disabilities. Federal Register July 30, 1993, Sec. 303.361;40968.
47. Ramey CT, Yeates KO, MacPhee D. Risk for retarded development among disadvantaged families: a systems theory approach to preventive intervention. Adv Special Educ 1984;4:249.
48. American Speech-Language-Hearing Association. The roles of speech-language pathologists in service delivery to infants, toddlers, and their families. ASHA 1990;32:4.
49. DEC Task Force on Recommended Practices. DEC Recommended Practices: Indicators of Quality Programs for Infants and Young Children with Special Needs and Their Families. Reston, VA: Council for Exceptional Children, 1993;47, 69.
50. Liptak GS. The role of the pediatrician in caring for children with developmental disabilities. Pediatr Ann 1995;24:232.

2

Causes of Developmental Delays and Disorders: Implications for Communication Competence

Frances P. Billeaud

As a preface to the materials included in this chapter, a brief discussion of terminology is in order. Terminology used by professionals who work with very young children who have or are at high risk for developmental delays and disorders can be somewhat confusing in that descriptors applied to conditions and behaviors have somewhat different meanings for different groups of professionals. It is important that practitioners not assume the definitions they are accustomed to using are understood or applied universally by other professionals working with the same child. Issues of terminology have been complicated further by the current societal trend to be "politically correct." Thus, the term *mental retardation* is customarily used by psychologists in defining limited mental capabilities and in applying diagnostic labels, whereas the individual who is so diagnosed or described by the psychologist may be labeled as *developmentally delayed* by teachers and other professionals who work in agencies serving persons with physical and mental disabilities. Persons who work in special education programs may refer to the same individual as *cognitively challenged* or *mentally handicapped* and may add a further qualification implying the degree to which the individual is affected (e.g., *mild-moderate* or *severe-profound*). Such labels are usually dictated by rules and regulations of governmental agencies, professional practice criteria, or by organizations devoted to serving selected groups of individuals with exceptionalities. Statutory language included in federal and state laws sometimes provides definitions that apply to eligibility for services, thus making use of particular terms imperative in qualifying individuals for the services to which only certain groups are entitled.

With those cautions in mind, this chapter provides information about infants and toddlers who exhibit a range of conditions or behaviors of concern to professionals. It is essential that practitioners recognize the status of a child who has been referred.

RECEIVING REFERRALS AND DETERMINING WHICH CHILDREN ARE AT RISK

Decisions about whether a given child is in need of treatment or management hinge on the child's condition or status in the eyes of the professional(s) to whom the referral has been made. Physicians look for specific physical conditions, disease processes, and anomalies that affect health or development. Psychologists and others look for identifiable behaviors, cognitive abilities, and indicators of mental and emotional status and development. Educators and early childhood development specialists look at child development across a number of "domains" (e.g., physical, social, self-help, cognitive) to make judgments about the child's readiness for instruction. Physical and occupational therapists evaluate the child's neuromotor maturation, physical capabilities, balance, use of concurrent sensory stimuli, and movement patterns. Speech-language pathologists (SLPs) assess sensory, oral neuromotor, qualitative and quantitative characteristics of the child's receptive and expressive communication, capabilities, and potential for development. Practitioners from other professional disciplines are trained to look at other aspects of the child's present levels of functioning and discern the probable potential for further developmental capabilities.

All professionals, each approaching his or her task from different perspectives based on training and experience, make decisions about a given child's status. They also make decisions as to whether interpretation of the data they have at their disposal suggests that the child's condition and behaviors represent one, or a combination, of the following possibilities:

- Difference: a condition or behavior that is somewhat unusual in certain circumstances but represents a variation of normal within the child's family, culture, or society (e.g., regional linguistic dialect patterns, short stature)
- Delay: a physical condition, state, or behavior having the potential to develop that is currently judged to be below expectations for the child's age, sex, or physical condition when measured against accepted norms or performance criteria. When no specific etiologic cause for late onset of language has been identified, such children are often said to be *language delayed*. Readers should note that the term *developmental delay* can be used by some groups to mean that the child continues to have, perhaps for a lifetime, the identified condition (e.g., pervasive developmental delay, mental retardation).
- Disorder: a condition or behavior that impairs functional abilities in one or more areas of development (e.g., language disorder, autistic spectrum disorder). Some disorders can be remediated, whereas others require development of compensatory skills, and still others can continue to exist despite all habilitative or rehabilitative efforts.
- Deficit: an identified absence or significant limitation in a specified physical attribute, function, or skill. Readers should note that the term

deficit is used by some professionals in the same way *developmental delay* is used by colleagues in other professional disciplines. For example, *mental retardation* implies that there is a lifelong deficit in cognitive ability. Optimized functioning of the individual with that condition can occur with early intervention and continued specialized training, but there will always be a deficit. Proponents of using the alternate term *developmental delay* recognize the presence of cognitive limitations but assert that it is unwise to use terminology that implies there is little prospect for improved functional abilities among affected individuals.

- Disability: a limitation in the ability to perform certain tasks in a typical manner (e.g., learning disability, language disability). The implication is that with proper assistance, alternative or adaptive methods can be employed to compensate for the condition that underlies the disability, allowing the affected individual to achieve a level of functional competence. Caution: Readers should note that *disability* is sometimes used, especially among nonprofessionals, interchangeably with the term *handicap*.
- Handicap: the degree to which an impaired condition or behavior prevents the affected person from engaging in life activities appropriate to others of the same age. What comprises a handicap for one person or situation may not do so for another. For example, unilateral vocal cord paralysis or developmental verbal dyspraxia would be a handicap for the respective purposes of singing or developing a "normal" speaking voice or articulation, but would not necessarily affect successful communication by competent users of augmentative communication devices or alternative strategies. Profound deafness, on the other hand, constitutes a continuing handicap across a variety of situations for affected individuals.

The Goal: Promoting Functional Abilities of Infants and Toddlers

Functional abilities of the developing child are affected by many factors, including congenital (present at birth) and acquired conditions and disorders. Among the common problems encountered by the SLP in work with the infant-toddler population are those related to (1) disease processes, (2) conditions (e.g., cerebral palsy), (3) structural anomalies (e.g., craniofacial clefting), (4) syndromes (collections of symptoms that are identifiable with specific genetic, chromosomal, physical, or psychoneurologic disorders), (5) sequences (a connected series of *conditions,* such as CHARGE sequence), (6) spectrum disorders (an array of *symptoms* related to a specifically diagnosed condition that can be predictive of a favorable prognosis or one that is less favorable, such as autistic spectrum disorder), and (7) physical or psychological trauma.

As was pointed out in Chapter 1, early intervention has the advantage of being applied at a time when the child's biological development is characterized by rapid proliferation of synaptic connections in the brain. Although that process does not overcome severe physical impairments (e.g., cerebral palsy) or correct anatomic anomalies (e.g., palatal clefts), it does optimize the neurophysiologic ecological environment in which habilitation can occur.

In terms of language development, "[t]he differential growth of the cortex of the cerebral hemispheres is of vital importance for speech and language function because the majority of neural structures for communication are integrated there . . . The cortical association areas lag behind the development of the cortical receptor areas that are present and active at birth" (p. 257).[1] Further, as Love and Webb point out,

[a]t 1 year the normal child has a vocabulary of one or more word approximations, usually names for objects that have been seen and sometimes touched. This stage of language development requires the ability to mix neural information from the auditory, somesthetic, and visual association areas. . . . The rapid growth of vocabulary in the second and third years of life . . . may well be a correlate of the maturation of [the] significant posterior association area in the parietal lobe, which combines information from surrounding association areas (p. 258).[1]

Because of the "plasticity" of the brain in the early years of life, when the very young child's brain is known to have been damaged, undamaged areas sometimes are capable of assuming the respective function(s) of the damaged area(s).[1] Hence, early maturation and growth of the brain itself work in favor of early-intervention efforts.

Appropriate early-intervention practices take into account environmental influences that support and are likely to promote positive developmental outcomes. Ideally, those practices are family focused, culturally sensitive, and specific to the child's needs.

The Concept of Prevention

As Wetherby and Prizant pointed out,

[e]arly identification of communication and language problems and appropriate intervention can prevent a number of difficulties that may be closely related to, and may possibly result from, early language and communication disorders. Although many questions remain regarding causal relationships, most investigators agree that infants and toddlers with communication delays or disorders are at high risk for the development of emotional and behavioral disorders . . . (p. 290).[2]

Prevention is a term that is frequently used in medical practices and other health care settings in a slightly different context than is usually applied by the general public. In the arena of health care, separate forms of prevention are recognized.

- *Primary prevention* is comprised of measures taken to prevent the occurrence of an undesirable outcome (e.g., genetic counseling that results in a couple's decision not to bear a child because the risk of a particular problem is considered too high).
- *Secondary prevention* consists of curing or ameliorating a problem that has occurred (e.g., surgical procedures employed to close a palatal cleft, install a cochlear implant, or clip a short lingual frenum; conducting speech-language therapy when full habilitation or rehabilitation is the goal).
- *Tertiary prevention* is reducing the negative effects of a given condition through treatment if amelioration of the condition is not possible (e.g., prescribing pharmacologic products to reduce or eliminate seizures, conducting speech-language therapy when compensatory skills are the goal, fitting appropriate amplification devices to optimize hearing in the presence of a known hearing loss).

Screening, Evaluation, Diagnosis, and Assessment

The causes of problems in communicative development are sometimes identifiable but often are not. It is highly desirable that the causes, if they can be identified, be understood, because the treatment or management plans for a given condition can differ from appropriate plans for other conditions. For example, the management approach for a child with a profound hearing loss is different from the one used for a child whose hearing is known to be within normal limits. Likewise, a child diagnosed with a particular syndrome or spectrum disorder is likely to benefit from a treatment-management plan designed to address the functional components affected by the cluster of characteristics associated with the syndrome or sequence. For example, management options for a child diagnosed with autism are quite different from those designed to optimize communication function in a child diagnosed with Down syndrome or Usher's syndrome.

Rubin[3] emphasized the importance of an accurate etiologic diagnosis:

> For the scientific community, the pursuit of an accurate etiological diagnosis aids the understanding of pathological mechanisms and hence the prevention of specific conditions (e.g., congenital infections, perinatal asphyxia, lead toxicity). Knowledge and understanding of etiology also allows for a greater appreciation of the manifestations of each condition when anticipating medical, therapeutic, and educational needs (pp. 25–26).

He noted, however, that the process of obtaining an accurate diagnosis is not always easy, may take time, and may in fact be elusive.

As pointed out above, terminology used in identifying children in need of further assessment varies across professional disciplines. Almost all practitioners agree that screening is the first level of identification. Screening can be formalized (i.e., specific protocols and criteria are applied to select a subgroup that meets the criteria for further assessment). Screening can also be informal (e.g., a family member or caregiver may sense that a child's behaviors or abilities are "different" from those of peers). Hearing screenings, cholesterol screenings, and lead-exposure screenings are common types of formal screenings with which almost everyone is familiar. Once a subgroup or individual of concern has been identified, the next level of investigation can involve assessment or evaluation of functional abilities or can move directly to the level of diagnosis.

A possible complication in arriving at a common understanding of the term *diagnosis* has to do with the level of confidence with which a particular diagnosis is invested. Technically, a diagnosis can be any one of the following: confirmed, differential, or definitive (most reliable); presumptive (highly probable on the basis of symptoms and testing conducted); or descriptive (implies the presence of a specific condition or set of behaviors with a commonly used label without actually confirming its presence by scientific means). Each of the diagnostic levels has practical applications, but each also has certain limitations. For example, a confirmed or differential diagnosis meets criteria for a specific label (e.g., acquired immunodeficiency syndrome, fragile X, sensorineural hearing loss) but fails to delineate expectations for functional abilities of the individual child diagnosed with the condition or disease. Such a diagnosis, however, is associated with general expectations with respect to probable response levels, behaviors, and prognosis.

Generally speaking, it is worth the effort to get as refined a diagnosis as possible, so that the implications of the condition or disease are well understood and treatment and management plans can be appropriately designed. Additionally, early diagnosis is a strong protective factor for prevention of secondary disabilities that often ensue. Superneau's statement in this regard could be applied to any disorder and is not exclusive to fetal alcohol syndrome (FAS) and fetal alcohol effects (FAE): "The early and appropriate diagnosis of FAS and FAE should be made to enhance the long-term outcome and reduce the disabilities experienced by affected individuals and their families."[4]

It is possible that a definitive or differential diagnosis requires documentation of characteristics that emerge over a period of several months or years, because many conditions derive from a failure of development or a disruption in developmental processes that typically proceed in an orderly and predictable manner. Cerebral palsy and autism are two examples of conditions that become evident with the passage of time.

The process of assessment of conditions and functions, however, is an ongoing process. It is crucial to the concepts of prevention and the benefits of early intervention. The recognition of atypical characteristics and functions as they emerge in the child's development can signal the need for specific management strategies to optimize development before a definitive diagnosis of a specific condition. Assessment procedures and tools are discussed in Chapters 6 and 7.

There is a certain level of tension between proponents of the so-called *medical model* of viewing atypical development and proponents of the so-called *developmental model*. On the one hand, it is argued that the medical model is based on identifying "deficits" and labeling children with terms that have negative implications, thus increasing the difficulties with which such children and their families must contend. The developmental model, on the other hand, identifies strengths and needs at given points of development and hence provides a more positive approach that is "family friendly." In truth, both models are useful and need not be mutually exclusive. Parents can choose to disclose a diagnostic "label" or keep it confidential; some individuals with whom the family comes in contact have a negative reaction to a child who is "different," no matter how unfair that attitude may be. Insensitivity is impossible to avoid, but it is not universal. Practitioners should know both the array of causes of atypical development *and* be competent in assessing current and potential skills and methods of facilitating optimal outcomes. Such competencies require working in collaboration with families and members of the professional community. Tracking developmental outcomes across individuals and diagnostic groups is an important responsibility of professionals who work with the infant and toddler population.

Because the lives of increasing numbers of very small, very sick infants are being saved in neonatal care facilities, and because those children are being seen increasingly in early intervention practices and preschool settings, it is also important that their progress be monitored and documented carefully so that improved prognoses for children with like problems can be formulated for the future. The following sections of this chapter are devoted to exploring specific factors that can cause a child to have a delay or disorder in development of communication and how those factors are identified. Chapter 7 provides more detailed information about assessing common effects of those factors on early communicative development.

CAUSES OF COMMUNICATIVE DISORDERS

Genetic and Chromosomal Aberrations

One method of discovering causes of disorders of human development is the application of knowledge in human genetics. Genetic and chromosomal problems associated with communicative disorders have become the focus of many professionals who specialize in the practice of medical speech pathology. Many, but not all, genetic and chromosomal problems are evident at or before birth and are often associated with a set of specific biological characteristics (phenotypes). Medical geneticists and SLPs have a natural alliance in following the course of infants and toddlers diagnosed with such disorders.

Because many children with chromosomal or genetic anomalies were doomed to early death until recent advances in medical technology improved the outlook, the literature on long-term outcomes for such children is limited and may, in fact, be unreliable in many instances. Now that more of these children are surviving and receiving early-intervention management from teams of professionals, it is becoming evident that the quality of life they can access, along with a more favorable outlook for developing functional abilities, can result in improved prognoses for many of them. Careful documentation of developmental outcomes among affected children is crucial to establishing more appropriate predictions of what other children diagnosed with the same disorders can achieve. Such information is critical to parental decision making and to the process of genetic counseling.

Congenital Anomalies, Syndromes, Sequences, Spectrum Disorders

Chapter 3 provides information about congenital syndromes and conditions associated with communicative disorders. It also includes a table showing common communicative disorders associated with recognized syndromes (see Table 3.5). Although the relative frequency of occurrence of all syndromes is quite small, a significant number of affected children are referred to communicative-disorders specialists. Bearing in mind that children with syndromes are first and foremost children who have the same needs of all children, those who are born with identified syndromes comprise a group whose treatment plans must address additional, and usually very specific, elements related to the characteristics of the specific syndrome(s) involved.

Recent discoveries have verified that chromosomal problems seen in affected individuals are somewhat variable even when the same chromosome is affected. This is so because the aberration on a given chromosome can occur at differing locations and can have different configurations (e.g., breaks, extra material, deletions, distortions), producing different effects. The important thing to remember is that not all persons with an identified chromosomal aberration have the same traits. Ongoing scientific research seeks to reveal specific sites with which particular traits are associated. Certain syndromes have already been "mapped." Clinical descriptions of characteristics and behaviors of individuals with such problems are urgently needed and are beginning to appear in the professional literature with increasing frequency.[5]

Other Diseases and Conditions Associated with Communicative Disorders

Acquired Diseases

Any disease that has the potential to affect cognition or central nervous system functioning has the potential to have an adverse effect on communicative development and function. Table 2.1 lists some of the more commonly encountered acquired diseases that can have a negative impact on communicative development.

Table 2.1 Etiologies Associated with Communicative Delays and Disorders

Allergies (especially those that are chronic and affect the respiratory system or mucosal tissues of the mouth, nose, and throat)

Asphyxia and extended or repeated episodes of hypoxia

Chronic illnesses resulting in persistent depressed energy and attentional levels

Congenital infections, diseases, or conditions
    Cytomegalovirus
    Encephalitis, meningitis
    Fetal alcohol effects
    Herpes
    Human immunodeficiency virus and acquired immunodeficiency syndrome
    Rh incompatibility (untreated)
    Rubella (German measles)
    Syphilis
    Toxoplasmosis
    Other

Other diseases and structural anomalies of the speech mechanism
    Choanal atresia
    Laryngeal papillomas
    Laryngeal stridor
    Laryngeal web
    Macroglossia
    Polyps

Physical anomalies (related to disorders of language)
    Brain anomalies
        Agenesis of the corpus callosum
        Anencephaly
        Encephalocele
        Holoprosencephaly
        Hydrocephaly
        Intraventricular hemorrhage
        Seizure disorders
        Stroke

    Other central nervous system anomalies and conditions
        Cerebral palsy
        Hypotonia (floppiness)

Physical injury and trauma
    Congenital, perinatal, in later infancy, and early childhood
    Accidents resulting in damage to physical mechanisms involved in understanding and producing language and speech
    Extended periods of intubation
    Injuries resulting from repeated intubation
    Radical surgical interventions required to treat injuries, diseases, and anomalies resulting in damage to mechanisms involved in understanding and producing speech and language
    Tracheostomy

Table 2.1 (continued)

Psychoemotional disorders
  See Table 2.2
  Attentional disorders*
    Attention deficit disorder
    Attention deficit hyperactivity disorder

Sensory impairment
  Hearing (congenital, acquired)
  Other sensory impairments (vision, balance, hypersensitivity to sensory stimuli)

Side effects or reactions to drugs or sera
  Allergies to components of the drug, suspension, or coating agents used in its delivery
  Ototoxic drugs
  Reactions to components of serum injections resulting in catastrophic effects

Syndromes
  See Table 3.5 for comprehensive details

*Although these disorders are classified as psychogenic in the *Diagnostic and Statistical Manual (4th ed)*, and other standard references, evidence exists that these conditions are actually neurogenic.

Trauma

Infants and toddlers are subject to physical trauma from the prenatal period through all stages of development during childhood. Damage to the respiratory system, the central nervous system, and to anatomic structures of the speech mechanism can occur as a result of mechanical pressures experienced by the fetus in the womb, adverse effects of treatment designed to preserve life (e.g., use of ototoxic drugs), or unanticipated problems at the time of delivery (e.g., damage caused by surgical instruments). Other factors that can occur at any time include surgical trauma (e.g., removal of malignancies requiring resections of adjacent structures involved in speech production or language development, inadvertent severing of a branch of the vagus nerve during surgical procedures unrelated to the speech mechanism), mechanical trauma (e.g., gunshot wounds to crucial organs, "shaken baby" syndrome), and other injuries incurred as a result of events such as near drowning, automobile accidents, and falls.

Infants and toddlers who require tracheostomies are of particular interest for a number of reasons. Simon and McGowen stated that tracheostomies in infants can be indicated for babies who are ventilator dependent and who have subglottic stenosis (narrowing of the airway below the glottis), tracheomalacia (softening of the tracheal cartilage), neuromuscular disorders, congenital anomalies (e.g., craniofacial anomalies, laryngeal neoplasms, cardiac anomalies, croup), and epiglottitis (inflammation of the epiglottis). They observed that, "[t]he development of speech and language in the tracheostomized child has been found to be related to the time of cannulation. If the child receives a tracheostomy during the prelinguistic stage of development . . . the speech and language therapy may be needed for both the establishment of a communication system and for early vocal production." (p. 1)[6]

Other types of trauma can lead to residual effects that impair speech or language development. This category includes such things as extensive scar tissue resulting from electrical burns to the oral structures (e.g., incurred when a child bites into a connected electrical cord), scar tissue residual to chemical burns (e.g., seen in children who swallow drain cleaners), and deleterious effects on the nervous system from exposure to heavy metals such as lead (which may be contained in paint chips ingested by children).

Regulatory, Emotional, and Mental Health Problems

Regulatory disorders in neonates are discussed in some detail in Chapter 5, but such problems are not limited to newborns. Children who are difficult to please and who seem "out of sorts" most of the time are exhibiting hypersensitivity to the requirements of adjusting to the demands of daily living and exhibiting that difficulty as behaviors that are described as "fussy" or "irritable." Such children may experience unsatisfactory interactions with their caregivers. As DeGangi and colleagues indicated,

> [c]hildren who are fussy, irritable, and demanding are extremely challenging for parents. Often parents cope by developing interaction patterns of understimulation or overstimulation. For example, parents who must often soothe and regulate their distressed child may find that they tend to retreat or shrink from interaction when their child is happy and to be content to "not rock the boat." In the case of the highly distractible child who appears to seek constant novelty, the parents may exacerbate the problem by presenting many activities or toys to their child to try to keep him or her happy (p. 115).[7]

Diagnosis of specific psychosocial or psychoemotional disorders is rare in children under the age of 3 years. However, a number of such problems have as part of their diagnostic criteria specified onset before age 3 years (e.g., autism). Clinical practitioners are encouraged to document persistent atypical behaviors in infants and toddlers that can lead to a subsequent diagnosis of attentional disorders, conduct disorders, and temperament and personality disorders, many of which have symptoms that appear in early childhood.

Post-traumatic stress disorder has been documented in children under the age of 3 years.[8-10] Such problems can manifest themselves as elective mutism and other types of speech problems that have a low rate of occurrence but are familiar to clinical practitioners (e.g., atypical stress, rate, fluency).

Landy and Peters commented about young children who exhibit excessively aggressive behavior:

> Delays of development in these children may be due primarily to neurologic or physiologic problems or to attachment disorders resulting from previous interactional difficulties. These problems may lead to difficulties

Table 2.2 Psychoemotional Disorders Having Known or Potential Association with Communicative Development

Attachment disorders
Childhood disintegrative disorder
Emotional disorders resulting from maltreatment, abuse, or neglect
Oppositional defiant disorder
Post-traumatic stress disorder
Separation defiant disorder
Pervasive developmental disorder
Autism
Asperger's syndrome
Landau-Kleffner syndrome
Pervasive developmental disorder, not otherwise specified

in interacting with others, delays in symbolization (such as language and pretend play), and failures in impulse control (p. 101).[11]

Table 2.2 lists an array of psychoemotional disorders that can be associated with difficulties in communicative development.

SINGLE AND MULTIPLE RISK FACTORS: THEIR ROLE IN DIAGNOSIS AND ASSESSMENT

Communicative disorders specialists must be aware of a variety of factors that place a child at risk for problems in developing speech and language. As Russell and Free observed, for example,

[c]hildren exposed to . . . potentially harmful substances [illegal substances and alcohol] during the vulnerable developmental period before birth often grow up in a childhood environment where the mother continues to abuse drugs and where there are limited mother-child interactions and learning experiences, placing the infant at both biological and environmental risk (p. 181).[12]

Preterm delivery per se is not a reliable predictor of developmental delays or disorders. However, preterm infants as a group, especially the subgroup in which neonatal complications are known to have occurred, are at risk for developmental difficulties. Hack and colleagues observed that neonatologists are saving 34% of infants of less than 751 g birthweight, 66% of those between 751 and 1,000 g, 87% of those weighing 1,001–1,250 g, and 93% at 1,251–1,500 g. "By obstetric measures of gestation, survival was 23% at 23 weeks, 34% at 24 weeks, and 54%

at 25 weeks" (p. 587).[13] Because many of these children develop severe intracranial abnormalities, it is estimated that 60% of those who do will have handicaps. Severe handicaps are found among 50% of infants born at 23 weeks, 38% of those born at 24 weeks, and 8% for those born at 25 weeks.[14] Ruff and Lawson observed that preterm babies with low birth weight observed at play at 9 months and 24 months exhibited less focused attention, lower levels of response to novel objects, and less reactivity than their full-term peers. They concluded that

> [t]hese data suggest that measures of attention may be important indicators of a child's present and future functioning. A child who engages in relatively little focused attention and exploration of objects in the latter half of the first year may learn less about objects and their properties and at the same time develop fewer strategies for gathering more information. The consequences could be serious for developing knowledge of the world and for emerging language (p. 122).[15]

The presence of one or more risk factors is not in and of itself predictive of atypical communicative development but indicates to the practitioner that the child may have a greater likelihood than other children of experiencing such difficulties. Even the indirect effects of some conditions, in areas seemingly unrelated to communication skills, can contribute to the confounding of atypical language and speech development. For example, lack of normal childhood experiences, which can be related to unusual child-rearing practices, can affect vocabulary acquisition or the child's level of curiosity, thus discouraging attempts to communicate. A family's overprotectiveness at one extreme or neglect at the other can discourage the child's desire to communicate. Impaired development of fine-motor skills, which are usually thought of as the province of occupational therapy, can have a counterpart in developmental dyspraxia of speech, a condition related to delayed and disordered speech in young children.

The SLP must be sensitive to all possible implications of information provided by the family or other knowledgeable informants when the case history is provided. It is sometimes the case that a combination of factors, rather than a single element, is the cause of a communication delay or disorder. Risk factors may reflect circumstances that were once operative in the child's life but no longer exist or, conversely, may be ongoing influences that may or may not be amenable to modification as part of the therapy program. An overview of causes of communicative disorders in infants and toddlers is provided in Table 2.3. Potential effects associated with specific conditions are listed in Table 2.4. Obviously the process of differential diagnosis dictates the direction of appropriate management, including referral and treatment options.

If atypical development is displayed, professionals are expected to untangle the "mysteries" with which they are presented when a family entrusts their child

Table 2.3 Overview of Causes of Communicative Disorders in Infants and Toddlers

Category and Onset	Examples of Diagnoses	Comment
Inherited disorders and syndromes Time of onset: conception	Down syndrome Goldenhar's syndrome Usher's syndrome	See Chapter 3 for detailed discussion.
Acquired diseases and disorders Time of onset: can occur pre-, peri-, or postnatally	Fetal alcohol syndrome Encephalitis Toxoplasmosis Papillomatosis Hearing loss resulting from ototoxic drugs	This category covers a broad range of viral, bacterial, and teratogenic etiologies.
Disruptions of growth in utero producing anomalies of structures or systems crucial to language and speech development Time of onset: prenatal	Certain forms of facial clefting Branchial arch deformities Anencephaly Laryngeal stridor Laryngeal web	Effects can range from conditions not clinically significant regarding communication (e.g., amniotic band syndrome affecting an extremity) to those that are crucial to communication development.
Sensory impairments Time of onset: usually prenatal but can occur in peri- or postnatal periods	Congenital or acquired hearing loss Multiple sensory impairments Extreme hyper- or hypo-sensitivity	Sensory impairments can result from congenital conditions or be acquired as a result of trauma, illness, or drug reactions.
Physical injury and trauma associated with conditions related to communicative development Time of onset: can occur pre-, peri-, or postnatally	Cerebral palsy Shaken baby syndrome Prolonged intubation Chemical burns affecting the speech mechanism Paresis or paralysis of one or both vocal cords	Physical injury and trauma can occur accidentally or result from surgical procedures or intentional physical abuse.
Severe or prolonged emotional trauma Time of onset: postnatal	Post-traumatic stress disorder Child abuse and neglect	The prevalence of child neglect and abuse is reportedly higher among children with developmental delays.
Disorders associated with global developmental delays and disorders Time of onset: prenatal or postnatal	Lead poisoning Certain metabolic disorders Failure to thrive	This category encompasses a wide range of possible problems.

Category and Onset	Examples of Diagnoses	Comment
Psychogenic disorders Time of onset: can be present but undetected at birth or appear in early childhood	Autism Pervasive developmental disorder not otherwise specified Childhood disintegrative disorder	Differential diagnosis is essential to selection of appropriate treatment options.
Delays and disorders arising from socioenvironmental factors Time of onset: variable	Extreme poverty coupled with low maternal educational level Extreme isolation and lack of stimulation	The factors noted have multiple effects that can involve poor nutrition and housing, immediate surroundings in which toxic particles are plentiful, lack of access to basic health care with consequent complications from common childhood diseases, lack of availability of appropriate speech-language models, and atypical child rearing practices.
Other neurophysiologic factors known to have a high co-occurrence of language development disorders Time of onset: variable	Attention deficit hyperactivity disorder Central auditory processing disorder Sensory integration disorder Learning disability	Many of the neurophysiologic mechanisms underlying these disorders are thought to be common to those underlying communicative functions. The effects of variable attention or atypical learning styles are likely to be disruptive of normal acquisition of selected language functions.

Table 2.4 Communicative Disorders and Related Conditions

Condition	Occurrence	Variable Effects
Speech or language impairments	20.8% of disabled school-age children have speech or language impairments. 3–10% of the general population have speech or language impairments.	Misarticulation Disorders of phonation Fluency disorders Receptive and expressive language disorders Occurrences shown are for primary speech or language disorders; such disorders often occur as part of other conditions and syndromes.
Hearing impairments	1:1,000 children is born with congenital deafness. Up to 5% of children from 0–18 years of age have hearing impairments. 1.3% of disabled 6–21 year olds have hearing loss. 1% of the general population are affected; 0.2% have severe losses.	Conductive hearing loss Sensorineural hearing loss Mixed hearing loss Deafness Condition can be acquired or congenital. Delayed or disordered speech and language commonly occur.
Developmental delay	2–5% of children under the age of 5 years have developmental delay.	Delays are frequently observed in the area of communication development in isolation or in combination with generalized delays across modalities.
Autism	15:10,000 children are affected. 0.5% of disabled 6–21 year olds are affected. Autism affects 0.5% of the population when combined with figures for pervasive developmental disorder.	Severely impaired language Idiosyncratic behaviors Disorders of social interaction
Multiple disabilities	1.8% of disabled 6–21 year olds have multiple disabilities.	Many multiple disabilities involve communicative disorders as a feature.
Traumatic brain injury	0.1% of disabled 6–21 year olds have traumatic brain injury.	Many children with traumatic brain injury experience communication problems.
Specific learning disabilities	51.1% of disabled 6–21 year olds have specific learning disabilities.	

Condition	Occurrence	Variable Effects
	70–80% of learning-disabled children have language disorders.	Note that the federal definition of dyslexia includes any problem with reading, writing, listening, or speaking.
Attention deficit disorder	2.2% of disabled 6–21 year olds have attention deficit disorder.	A large number of children with attentional disorders also have language delays and disorders. Attention deficit hyperactivity disorder can be diagnosed in some children before the age 3 years.
Cerebral palsy	3–7% of all live births have cerebral palsy. 0.5% of the general population are affected.	Cerebral palsy is diagnosed before the age of 3 years. Up to 50% of children with cerebral palsy have communicative disorders.

to the professionals' care. In addition to comparing the child's development to normative expectations, the SLP considers at least two other sources of information: (1) reports from others who have cared for the child and family and (2) completion of a thorough case history that explores an array of information the SLP finds indispensable to understanding a given child's situation. Examples of formats for documenting more detailed or supplementary case-history information specific to identifying risk factors and family histories that are useful in determining when to refer families for genetic consultations are provided in Appendix A.

The potential for delayed or disordered communicative development inferred from the presence of single or multiple risk factors must be ascertained. Practitioners take into account prenatal, perinatal, and postnatal events and conditions; family history; environmental risks and adverse societal conditions; infant temperament and capacity for self-regulation regarding formation of attachments; and the emotional stability of the child. Reliable conclusions can be drawn only after balancing the known risks with known protective factors such as family stability, a secure and nurturing environment, physical health, cognitive ability, and emotional health.

It is not always possible to obtain a confirmed diagnosis, especially in very young children. In such cases, it is the presence or absence of one or more risk factors that may lead the practitioner in the direction of a presumptive diagnosis, on which the selection of management or intervention strategies is based. In many situations, it is essential that a team of professionals work alongside the parents in identifying the parameters of the problem(s) at hand and in devising optimal care and management plans. Chapter 4 addresses the concept of teams and processes of effective team operations.

REFERENCES

1. Love RJ, Webb WG. Neurology for the Speech-Language Pathologist (3rd ed). Boston: Butterworth–Heinemann, 1996.
2. Wetherby AM, Prizant BM. Toward Earlier Identification of Communication and Language Problems in Infants and Young Children. In SJ Meisels, E Fenichel (eds), New Visions for the Developmental Assessment for Infants, Toddlers, and Young Children. Washington, DC: Zero to Three/National Center for Infants, Toddlers, and Families, 1993;289.
3. Rubin IL. Etiology of developmental disabilities. Infants Young Child 1990;3:25.
4. Superneau D. Fetal Alcohol Syndrome and Fetal Alcohol Effects: Clues to Detection and Behavioral Implications. Presentation at the Contemporary Forums Conference on The Child with Special Needs, New Orleans, LA, April 1997.
5. Weistuch L, Schiff-Myers NB. Research note: chromosomal translocation in a child with SLI and apraxia. J Speech Hear Res 1996;39:668.
6. Simon BM, McGowan JS. Tracheostomy in young children: implications for assessment and treatment of communication and feeding disorders. Infants Young Child 1989;1:1.
7. DeGangi GA, Craft P, Castellan J. Treatment of sensory, emotional, and attentional problems in regulatory disordered infants: parts 1 and 2. Infants Young Child 1991;3:1, 9.
8. Zeanah CH. The Assessment and Treatment of Infants and Toddlers Exposed to Violence. In JD Osofsky, E Fenichel (eds), Caring for Infants and Toddlers in Violent Environments: Hurt, Healing, and Hope. Arlington, VA: Zero to Three/National Center for Clinical Infant Programs, 1994;29.
9. Zeanah CH, Boris N, Scheeringa M. Psychopathology in infancy. J Child Psychol Psychiatry 1997;38:81.
10. Zeanah CH. Disorders of Attachment. Paper presented at the Contemporary Forums Conference on The Child with Special Needs, New Orleans, LA, April 1997.
11. Landy S, Peters RD. Identifying and treating aggressive preschoolers. Infants Young Child 1990;3:78.
12. Russell FF, Free TA. Early intervention for infants and toddlers with prenatal drug exposure. Infants Young Child 1992;3:78.
13. Hack M, Horbor JD, Malloy MH, et al. Very low birth weight outcomes of the National Institute of Child Health and Human Development Neonatal Network. Pediatrics 1991;87:587.
14. Allen M, Donohue P, Dusman A. The limit of viability: neonatal outcome of infants born at 22–25 weeks gestation. N Engl J Med 1993;329:1597.
15. Ruff HA, Lawson KR. Assessment of Infants' Attention During Play with Objects. In CE Schaefer, K Gitlin, A Sandgrund (eds), Play Diagnosis and Assessment. New York: Wiley, 1991;115.

3

Selected Medical Aspects of Communication Disorders

Theodore F. Thurmon and Suzanne Greenwood Thurmon

The medical aspects of communication disorders can be either acquired or congenital in nature. In both categories, it is necessary to establish the presence of speech and language deficits and to assess capabilities by testing. Deficits and capabilities can vary widely within diagnostic categories. Acquired disorders usually result from injury (e.g., trauma, infection, toxins). Their mechanisms can be better understood when it is possible to confer with the physician who evaluated or treated the injury.

Focal lesions of the central nervous system, peripheral nerves, and the organs of articulation can produce specific speech and language disorders (Figure 3.1). It is easy to see how trauma or infection can destroy any of these structures, but some toxins have focal effects also. Aminoglycoside antibiotics (e.g., gentamicin, kanamycin, neomycin, streptomycin, tobramycin) have a specific eighth nerve toxicity in persons who are genetically predisposed to this effect. The cochlea and retina are exquisitely sensitive to anoxia and noxious agents.

Asphyxia, such as that which complicates some births, also produces a cognitive defect because of general brain injury. Many noxious agents also result in generalized brain injury. Equivalent degrees of brain malfunction can also result from poor brain formation or microcephaly, which is typical of Down syndrome and a number of other congenital disorders. Congenital microcephaly in progeny is the most frequently identified result of consanguineous matings in population isolates.

Congenital means that a disorder is present at birth but not due to events complicating the birth. Congenital disorders are the focus of this section. Although present, such disorders may not be noticed at birth but may become evident as the child grows older. These various disorders have little in common and can be understood only through study of the individual disorders.

EFFECTS OF TERATOGENS

Congenital disorders are usually heritable, though, in rare cases, an injury to the developing fetus can result in a congenital disorder. Fetal injury, caused by teratogens, is much less frequent than is commonly thought. Few pregnan-

49

Locations

Levels: Structures; symptomatology

Level 5: Frontal lobes; stuttering

Level 4: Temporoparietal cortex; expressive and receptive aphasia

Level 3: Cerebellum; broken, monotone speech

Level 2: Corticobulbar tract; poorly coordinated speech

Level 1: Cranial nerves VII, X, XII; dysarthria, distortion

Figure 3.1 Locations of neurologic lesions and resulting speech and language disorders. (Adapted from FP Bakes. Speech, Language, and Hearing. In F Falkner [ed], Human Development. Philadelphia: Saunders, 1966.)

cies pass uneventfully, but the events rarely harm the fetus. That fact, combined with the difficulties of diagnosing heritable causes, leads to the frequent erroneous assumption of acquired disease or injury. There is also a time-honored tendency at all levels of society to turn to fantasy to explain our undesirable features.[1] The very word *teratogen* derives from a Greek term for importunate actions of the gods.

Table 3.1 is a list of known teratogens and their effects. Most of them must be delivered directly to the fetus in large doses in the first 10 weeks of gestation, if ill effects are to be realized. When this occurs, the degree of affectation of the fetus can vary because of heritable differences in defense mechanisms of the fetus (i.e., the same dose can produce severe defects in some fetuses and little or no effect in others). There is a potential for speech and language disorders in all patients who have visible effects of teratogens.

The impact of a teratogenic disorder on speech and language results either from damage to anatomic structures that are important to speech production and language development or from neurologic damage. Teratogens usually damage multiple areas at once, producing syndromes (*syn* = together, *drome* = run), in which anomalies of multiple structures occur together in a recurring association. Important remarks about syndromes follow the Common Heritable Anomalies section.

Table 3.1   Currently Characterized Human Teratogens

Medications

Direct Effects (Same as Postnatal)	*Teratogenic Effects (continued)*
Dependency-inducing drugs • Withdrawal	**Cocaine** • Limb, heart, and neural tube defects
Hormones and antihormones • Endocrine effects: developmental in fetus also	**Fluconazole** • Craniofacial and skeletal anomalies
Streptomycin, Daraprim, quinine • Deafness	**Hydantoins** • Wide face, nail hypoplasia, fingertip hypoplasia
Tetracyclines • Dental malformation	**Lithium** • Ebstein's anomaly of heart
Obstetric drugs • Fetus more sensitive	**Methyl mercury** • Deafness, blindness, paralysis
Delayed Effects	**Penicillamine** • Skin hyperelastosis
Diethylstilbestrol • Genital metaplasia	**Smoking** • Low birth weight
Teratogenic Effects	
Poor fetal growth and development are common to all	**Trimethadione** • V-shaped eyebrows, dental and palatal anomalies
Alcohol • Blepharophimosis, faint philtrum	**Thalidomide** • Phocomelia, heart malformation, deafness
Aminopterin • Dwarfism, hypoplastic cranium	**Valproic acid** • Brachycephaly, microstomia, spina bifida
Anticoagulants • Stippled epiphyses, hypoplastic nose	**Vitamin A cogeners** (retinoic acid) • Microtia, clefts, brain anomalies
Carbamazepine • Upslanting eyes, short nose, nail hypoplasia	

Infections

Maternal Infections	*Fetal Infections*
Defects result from focal thrombotic vascular occlusions in the fetus **Purulent infections** **Viral infections** **Amnionitis**	Low birth weight, vision and hearing defects, and mental retardation are common to all Cytomegalovirus Rubella Syphilis Toxoplasmosis Varicella

Table 3.1 (continued)

Maternal Disorders

Diabetes mellitus	**Myasthenia gravis**
• Conotruncal defects, caudal regression	• Newborn myasthenia
Hypertension	**Myotomic dystrophy**
• Low birth weight, microcephaly, PDA	• Arthrogryposis, mental retardation
Hyperthermia	**Phenylketonuria**
• Arthrogryposis, low birth weight, neural tube defect	• Microcephaly, dwarfism, prominent midface
Malnutrition	**Twinning**
• Low birth weight	• Disruption, sirenomelia, exstrophy of cloaca

Hazardous Procedures and Trauma

Maternal Trauma and Surgical Complications	*Direct Fetal Trauma*
Fetal cerebral blood flow cessation causes defects	**Hypertonic intravenous contrast material**
	• Focal thrombotic vascular occlusions
Maternal hypotension	**X-ray** (therapeutic or catastrophic, not diagnostic)
Maternal hypoxia	• Microcephaly, eye and genital malformation

Source: TF Thurmon. Medical Genetics Primer. Shreveport, LA: LSUMC-S Bookstore, 1997;10-9.

Fetal injury should not be accepted as the cause of a congenital disorder, except when there is forthright documentation of the actual injury. For example, the inherited disorder chorioretinal cerebral dysplasia[2] so closely mimics congenital toxoplasmosis that these disorders cannot be differentiated without accurate serologic testing. Nearly every other teratogenic disorder also has a genetic equivalent. This may seem to be of little consequence to the speech and language therapist, but greater comprehension of a problem comes from the understanding of its etiology. Assumptions about causation can be sharpened also. Hearing impairment arising from congenital toxoplasmosis infection is often said to be common; however, studies based on serologic diagnosis disclose that only about 2 of 1,000 newborns with serologic evidence of congenital toxoplasmosis infection have congenital hearing impairment.[3] In contrast, careful evaluation of families of cases of newborns with congenital hearing impairment discloses a heritable cause in at least 50%.[4]

COMMON HERITABLE ANOMALIES

A number of heritable anomalies that affect speech and language development are much more common than teratogenic disorders. They are most fre-

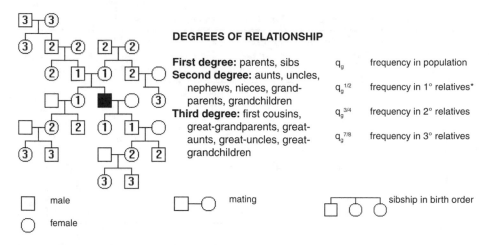

DEGREES OF RELATIONSHIP

First degree: parents, sibs
Second degree: aunts, uncles,
  nephews, nieces, grand-
  parents, grandchildren
Third degree: first cousins,
  great-grandparents, great-
  aunts, great-uncles, great-
  grandchildren

q_g	frequency in population
$q_g^{1/2}$	frequency in 1° relatives*
$q_g^{3/4}$	frequency in 2° relatives
$q_g^{7/8}$	frequency in 3° relatives

☐ male ◯ female ☐—◯ mating ☐◯◯ sibship in birth order

Figure 3.2 Calculation of frequencies of polygenic disorders among relatives of a patient. Numbers in the symbols represent degrees of relationships. The patient is represented by the darkened symbol. (*The notation is in fractional exponent, e.g., $q_g^{1/2} = \sqrt[2]{q_g}$. A frequency is a fraction; a fractional exponent of a fraction has a larger numerical value: If frequency is 1 in 10, or 0.1, the square root is 0.32, or 1 in 3.) (Adapted from TF Thurmon. Medical Genetics Primer. Shreveport, LA: LSUMC-S Bookstore, 1997.)

quently found as isolated defects in an otherwise normal person (nonsyndromic). These common heritable anomalies occur even more frequently among relatives of affected persons than in the general population; in fact, the frequency of such an anomaly among immediate family members is the square root of the population frequency.[5] Extensions of that mathematical relationship have developed the theory of polygenic inheritance. This theory holds that some traits are caused by the total effects of all genes and all environmental factors. The effects must be strong enough to produce a degree of the trait that can be perceived. There are gradations in the strengths of the effects above that level, so the trait has gradations from mild to severe. Though polygenic inheritance remains a theory, it allows differentiation from other etiologies and prediction of frequency with which a given disorder may occur in relatives. Figure 3.2 and Table 3.2 illustrate that concept.

Common heritable anomalies can affect speech and language functions through either anatomic or neurologic aberrations. Clefts of the lip or palate interfere with articulation and resonance. The same primordial structures of the embryo contribute to formation of both the heart and the organs of articulation. Hence, cleft palate and high-arched palate are often associated with heart malformation, as are middle- and inner-ear anomalies, retrognathia, glossoptosis, and laryngeal hypoplasia, any occurrence of which can adversely affect speech. Members of the immediate family may have similar disorders that are clinically

Table 3.2 Observed Frequencies of Polygenic Disorders among Relatives

Disorders	Normal Parents		Affected Parents	
	Population Frequency	Risk of Second Affected Child	Risk of Having an Affected Child	Risk of Second Affected Child
Clefts of lip or palate	0.1%	2%	NA	NA
Bilateral	NA	6%	NA	NA
Heart malformations	0.5%	2% (same type)	14% (if mother)	NA
Additional risk	NA	4% (other type)	NA	NA
Neural tube defects				
United States	0.1%	3.2%	4%	8%
United Kingdom	0.3%	5%	NA	NA

NA = statistically significant data not available.
Source: Adapted from CO Carter. Multifactorial Genetic Disease. In VA McKusick, R Claiborne (eds), Medical Genetics. New York: Hospital Practice Publishers, 1973.

evident. However, a more insidious problem is that parents may instead have milder forms such as velopharyngeal incompetence, and may thus prove to be poor role models for speech development (i.e., an affected child's speech defect may be in part a learned pattern).

The neural tube is an embryonic structure that, when projected onto the completely formed human, extends from the glabella at the nasal root to the coccyx at the base of the spine. The central nervous system and associated bony structures derive from the neural tube. Well-known anomalies of the neural tube include anencephaly, encephalocele, and myelomeningocele (spina bifida). Although these may appear to be localized, there is, in truth, aberrant development throughout the nervous system, and speech production and language development are often affected.

The tangible nature of these common heritable anomalies has facilitated the confirmation of their heritability. However, development of speech and language appears to also be heritable in the same manner (i.e., polygenic).[6] Well-known congenital disorders of speech and language, when occurring in an otherwise normal person, also affect family members in frequencies similar to those of the common heritable anomalies.[7] As with the common heritable anomalies, occurrence of a speech and language disorder in a parent complicates therapy.

Approximately 5 of 1,000 children have isolated, nonsyndromic, congenital mental deficiency (simple familial mental retardation) that is also polygenic.[4] Language deficit is the most significant problem among those children, and those with very poor mental functions may exhibit poor articulation skills as well. As with the common heritable anomalies, parents may have either the

Table 3.3 Isolated versus Syndromic Forms of Common Anomalies

Disorder	Isolated	Syndromic
Cleft lip	88%	12%
Cleft palate	60%	40%
Heart malformation	75%	25%
		(Half are chromosomal.)
Neural tube defects	90%	10%

Source: TF Thurmon. Medical Genetics Primer. Shreveport, LA: LSUMC-S Bookstore, 1997.

same or milder degrees of affectation that can contribute to learned speech aberrations and can lead to compliance problems in continuing therapy. Cultural language differences, also familial but not heritable, can coexist with these developmental disorders and confuse the diagnosis. Careful neurologic and developmental assessment may be required for differentiation.

IS IT AN ISOLATED PROBLEM OR IS IT PART OF A SYNDROME?

A major pitfall to the understanding of congenital disorders is the fact that, although they usually occur as isolated problems in otherwise normal persons, they are also found as a feature of various syndromes in other persons. For example, about half of cases of heritable hearing impairment have a syndrome instead of an isolated deficit.[4] Syndromes can have diverse causes, as well as many features other than those associated with speech and language impairment, so that all patients cannot be approached in the same way. Table 3.3 compares frequencies of isolated versus syndromic anomalies.

In general, persons with syndromes have more limited potentials than do persons with isolated defects. Some features of the syndromes can limit their ability to respond to speech and language therapy. Management requires a multidisciplinary approach. The practical difficulty of securing and coordinating multidisciplinary management is another limiting factor. Although some of the syndromes can be recognized on sight, diagnosis usually requires the services of an experienced physician such as a medical geneticist or a dysmorphologist. Table 3.4 illustrates the breadth of issues to be considered.

MENDELIAN DISORDERS

Mendelian disorders are those heritable disorders that have discrete inheritance (i.e., dominant, recessive, X-linked). The term *discrete* has a mathematical basis. It means that a person either has the gene or does not have the gene, and there are no gradations. Figures 3.3 through 3.6 illustrate mendelian inheritance patterns.[4]

Table 3.4 Examples of Syndromes Associated with Neural Tube Defects

Syndrome	Findings	Etiology
Goldenhar syndrome	Hemifacial microsomia, preauricular tags, epibulbar dermoid, microtia, hemivertebrae	Polygenic
Chromosome 18 trisomy	Gestational dwarfism, microcephaly, prominent occiput, small ears, small face, short sternum, overlap of index finger onto middle finger and little finger onto ring finger, contractures of hips and fingers, septal heart malformations	Chromosomal
Fetal valproate syndrome	Fetal flow heart malformations, neural tube defects, telecanthus, short nose, small mouth, long fingers	Teratogenic

Source: Adapted from KL Jones. Smith's Recognizable Patterns of Human Malformation (4th ed). Philadelphia: Saunders, 1988.

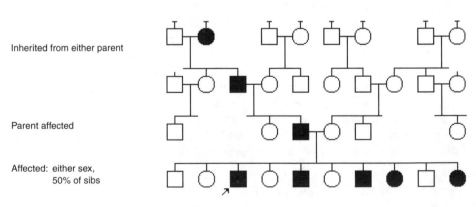

Figure 3.3 Autosomal dominant inheritance.

Parental consanguinity

Normal parents

Affected: either sex,
25% of sibs

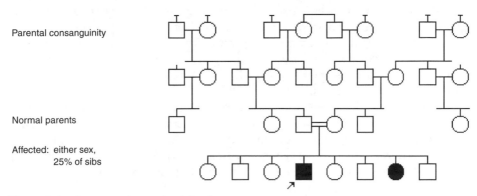

Figure 3.4 Autosomal recessive inheritance.

Female carriers = heterozygotes
Affected female: heterozygous
mother, hemizygous father

More frequent in males
No male-to-male transmission

Progeny of heterozygote:
50% of sons affected,
50% of daughters carriers

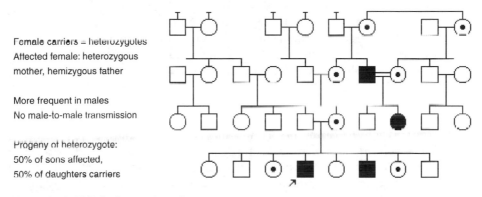

Figure 3.5 X-linked recessive inheritance.

More frequent in females
Milder in heterozygote
Homozygosity can be lethal

No male-to-male transmission
Hemizygosity can be lethal

Progeny of heterozygote:
50% affected, either sex

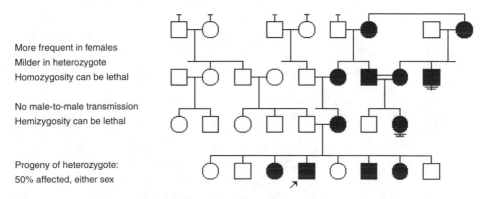

Figure 3.6 X-linked dominant inheritance.

A number of mendelian disorders (approximately 150 are known) produce speech and language deficits, and all are rare. They range from anatomic abnormalities to neurologic aberrations to specific disorders of speech and language. Some are isolated abnormalities, but most are syndromes. The best guide to mendelian disorders is the encyclopedic publication by McKusick[2] (Internet address: http://www3.ncbi.nlm.nih.gov/Omim/).

The isolated X-linked trait speech and language disorder with orofacial dyspraxia is characterized by an inability to generate syntactic rules for tense, number, and gender. Familial developmental dysphasia is an isolated autosomal dominant trait in which the development of spoken language is severely delayed. Isolated dyslexia 1 and dyslexia 2 are autosomal dominant disorders that entail language-based learning impairment.

Nonsyndromic hearing loss is one of the better-defined isolated mendelian traits.[8] Thirteen autosomal recessive forms are known at present. Most are prelingual (onset before language development) and stable. There are also 13 autosomal dominant forms, most of which are postlingual (onset after language development) and progressive. There are eight X-linked forms, two postlingual progressive, three prelingual stable, and three not yet fully defined.

Diagnosis of mendelian disorders usually requires the services of an experienced physician. However, these disorders are often present among relatives, and this can be discerned through genealogy evaluation. Even without a precise diagnosis, clinical expectations can be formulated for a new case by cataloguing the characteristics of other cases in the family. Public records of marriages, births, deaths, and successions are the most accurate sources of genealogic data, but recollections of family members are the most commonly used. The Catholic Church and the Mormon Church are also good sources of data and are frequently consulted by health professionals who specialize in diagnosing genetic disorders.

The most informative data are found among the descendants of the patient's great-grandparents and are often limited to a small section of the family's genealogy. There is a standardized manner of recording genealogic information that allows one to recognize inheritance patterns, providing sufficient family data exist. A genealogy chart is also a very compact representation of large amounts of family data. Charting conventions are variable, so a legend should be included with a given patient's chart. Figure 3.7 shows the standard charting method.

Parents of young children with heritable disorders may seek, or be advised to seek, information about the possibility that they may have other children with the same disorder, or they may be interested to know whether their affected child or siblings are likely to bear children with the same disorder. Such counseling should be provided by qualified health care professionals, such as medical geneticists and genetic counselors, to whom other practitioners can refer the family. Due to experience in handling the wide breadth of genetic disorders, the medical geneticist is also in a unique position to assist the speech and language

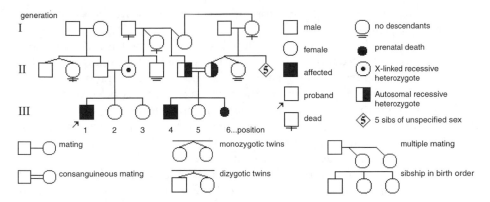

Figure 3.7 Guide to genealogy charting. (Adapted from TF Thurmon. Medical Genetics Primer. Shreveport, LA: LSUMC-S Bookstore, 1997.)

practitioner in coordination of the management of the more complex congenital disorders of speech and hearing.

FREQUENCIES OF DISORDERS

Among all of the categories and individual disorders discussed here, which are the common ones? There are at least two levels of answers to that question. (1) the perspective of the individual speech and language practitioners and (2) population frequency.

Many factors govern the actual frequencies at which individual disorders occur in a particular speech and language practice. For example, some speech and language practitioners are associated with a special interest group, such as a craniofacial surgery team. Disorders that are extremely rare, such as Apert's syndrome, can be seen frequently in such situations. Other categories of disorders may be treated by other special interest groups that do not ordinarily include a speech and language practitioner. Although those disorders may, in truth, be quite frequent and may frequently entail speech and language aberrations, they may not often come to the attention of the speech and language practitioner. Heart malformations are a good example of this type of disorder.

Many population frequency data have already been mentioned in the discussions of the individual disorders. Perhaps the most frequent individual disorder is Down syndrome, which occurs in 0.16% of newborns per year. Actual population prevalence is higher because modern medical care enables prolonged longevity of individuals with this syndrome. Heart malformations as a group are a bit more common than Down syndrome at birth, but individual types of heart malformations are less common. Cleft lip and palate, neural tube defects, deafness, nonsyndromic speech and language disorders, and nonsyndromic mental deficiency are a bit less common. Most other congenital disorders occur at low population frequencies.

The basal (lowest) frequency of an autosomal dominant mendelian disorder is the mutation rate, approximately 0.001%. For an autosomal recessive disorder, the basal figure can be smaller or larger, as it is a function of both mutation and the mating structure of the population. Various types of selection mechanisms result in polymorphisms of many mendelian disorders. A *polymorphism* is a situation in which a disorder occurs at a frequency that is higher than the basal rate. Some mendelian disorders can also attain high frequencies in specific population isolates due to genetic drift or selection.

Most teratogenic disorders are also quite rare. Only a few (i.e., fetal effects of alcohol, cytomegalovirus, tobacco) occur at frequencies above basal levels of autosomal dominant mendelian disorders. This is due, in part, to dose dependency, but surveillance and control have also played important parts in keeping these problems at bay. Surveillance and control mechanisms for teratogens will become increasingly important as our society develops more technological complexity.

Considering teratogenic and mendelian syndromes, those that affect speech and language number in the hundreds. All are rare, and relatively few have received any specific study of the speech and language component,[9] which points out the importance of diagnostic evaluation of each patient by the speech and language practitioner. Table 3.5 summarizes available data about the clinically recognizable syndromes that have had some study of the speech and language component.

An equal number of syndromes have had some study of the speech and language component but are recognizable only by the neurologist on the basis of a set of neurologic abnormalities in recurring association. Perhaps the most insidious of those disorders are the inborn errors of metabolism that can produce relatively few recognizable features and may not be known to exist unless laboratory testing has been done for them.[4] As they are all rare, laboratory testing may not be available through standard hospital and clinical laboratories. Help is often available from the medical geneticist, who can provide the tests or know where they can be obtained. Laboratory testing for these disorders should be considered in any patient in whom a plausible etiology of a speech or language disorder is lacking.

Table 3.5 Clinically Recognizable Syndromes That Have Had Some Study of the Speech and Language Component

Syndrome	CLP	NE	LI	A	C	R	V	CHL	SNL
Aarskog hypertelorism, brachydactyly, shawl scrotum				P	O				
Ablepharon macrostomia				F	F			F	P
Achondroplasia				O		F	F	F	
Acrodysostosis				F	F			O	
Acro-osteolysis				P	P			O	
ADAM fetal mutilation, constricting bands	F			F	F	F		F	
Albers-Schönberg osteopetrosis				F	F			F	F
Alport nephropathy and deafness									F
Alström deafness, retinitis pigmentosa, obesity, diabetes									F
Angelman jerky gait, large mouth, mental deficiency			F		F				
Aniridia, cerebellar ataxia, mental deficiency		F	F						
Apert acrocephaly, mitten syndactyly				F	F	F		F	
Beckwith-Wiedemann exomphalos, macroglossia, gigantism				F	F				
Bilateral femoral dysgenesis, unusual facies	F			F		F		F	
Binder maxillonasal dysplasia				O					
Bloom dwarfism, actinic dermatitis					O		F		
Branchio-oculofacial syndrome				F					
Carpenter acrocephalopolysyndactyly				F	F	F		F	
Cerebrocostomandibular syndrome			F	F					
Chondrodysplasia punctata (Conradi-Hünermann syndrome)				F				F	
Chromosome 10q+[a]				F		F			
Chromosome 11p+[a]				F		F	F		

Table 3.5 (continued)

Syndrome	CLP	NE	LI	A	C	R	V	CHL	SNL
Chromosome 18p–[a]			F	F	F				
Chromosome 18q–[a]	F		F	F	F	F		F	
Chromosome 1q+[a]	F		F	F	F	F		F	
Chromosome 21 trisomy (Down syndrome)[a]			F	F	F	O		F	I
Chromosome 3p+[a]	F		F	F	F	F		F	
Chromosome 4p–[a]	F		F		F	F		F	
Chromosome 4p+[a]			F		F				
Chromosome 5p– (cri du chat syndrome)[a]			F		F		F		
Chromosome 6q–[a]	F		F	F	F	F		F	
Chromosome 7q+[a]	F		F	F	F	F		F	
Chromosome 8 trisomy[a]			F	F	F				
Chromosome 9p–[a]			F		F				
Chromosome 9p+[a]	F		F		F	F		F	
Chromosome X– (Turner syndrome), short stature, sexual infantilism	O			O	I	O		F	F
Clasped thumb, mental retardation		F	F						
Clefting and oral teratoma	F			F	I	F		F	
Cockayne precocious senility			F	F	F	I	F	F	F
Coffin-Siris coarse face, hypoplastic fifth digits			F						
Cohen hypotonia, obesity, prominent incisors			F	P	F				
Costello faciocutaneoskeletal syndrome		F	F						
Crouzon craniofacial dysostosis				F	O	F		F	
Cryptophthalmia	O			O	O	O	O	F	F
de Lange synophrys, dwarfism, limb reduction	F		F	F	F	F	F	F	
Diastrophic dwarfism				O		F	F	F	
DiGeorge syndrome (CATCH-22)	F							F	

Syndrome	CLP	NE	LI	A	C	R	V	CHL	SNL
Dominant craniometaphyseal dysplasia				F		F		F	O
Dubowitz short asymmetric eye slits, eczema, short stature	O		F	P	F	O	F	O	
Dysautonomia		F		F	F	F	P		
Ectrodactyly, ectodermal dysplasia, cleft palate (EEC)	F			F	O	F		F	
Ehlers-Danlos hyperelasticity, fragile tissues				O				O	
Extrapyramidal disorder, hypogonadism, alopecia		F	F						
Facio-auriculo-vertebral sequence				F	O	F		F	
Fetal alcohol growth deficiency, microcephaly, blepharophimosis	F		F	F	F	F		F	
Floating-Harbor short stature, triangular face, language delay						F			
Fragile X large ears, long face, cluttering speech			F			F			
Freeman-Sheldon whistling face, ulnar deviation of hands				F		F		P	
Frontometaphyseal dysplasia								F	O
Frontonasal dysplasia	O			O	O	O		O	
Growth retardation, small puffy hands and feet, eczema		F	F						
Hall-Riggs mental retardation, depressed face, bone dysplasia			F						
Hallermann-Streiff microcephaly, small nose, hypotrichosis				P	F	O			
Hallervorden-Spatz late infantile neuro-axonal dystrophy		F	F						
Homocystinuria ectopia lentis, malar flush, osteoporosis		F	F	P	F	P			
Hydrocephalus, agyria, retinal dysplasia		F	F						
Hypochondroplasia				O	F	F		O	
Hypoglossia-hypodactyly	O			F		O		O	
Immune deficiency, centromeric instability, tongue protrusion			F	F					

Table 3.5   (continued)

Syndrome	CLP	NE	LI	A	C	R	V	CHL	SNL
Johanson-Blizzard hypoplastic alae nasi, hypothyroidism	F	F		F				F	
Kniest flat face, thick joints, platyspondyly, short stature	F			F		F		F	
Langer-Geidion trichorhinophalangeal syndrome			F		O			F	
Larsen flat face, joint luxations, short fingernails	F			F		F		F	
Leopard lentigines, hypertelorism, deafness, pulmonic stenosis					F				F
Macrocephaly, lipomas, hemangiomas			F		F				
Male pseudohermaphroditism, mental retardation (Verloes type)			F		F				F
Maxillofacial dysostosis		F		F					
Mental retardation, X-linked-6, gynecomastia, obesity[b]			F		F				
Mental retardation (Buenos Aires type)[c]			F		F				
Mesomelia-synostoses	F			F					
Moebius sequence of facial diplegia				F	F	F			
Mohr cleft tongue, deafness, bifid hallux (OFD II)	O			O	O	O		O	
Mulibrey nanism, pericardial constriction, retinal yellow dots					O		F	F	
Multiple synostoses								F	
Myasthenia, congenital, elongated face		F		F			F		
Myotonic dystrophy	O	F		F	F	F		O	
Myotonic myopathy, chondrodystrophy, oculofacial anomalies	F		F						
Nager acrofacial dysostosis				F	O	F		F	
Neurofibromatosis				O	O	O	O		O
Noonan pulmonic stenosis, webbed neck, short stature				F	F	I		O	
Norrie pseudoglioma of retina					F				F
Opitz hypertelorism, hypospadias (G, BBB)	F			F	O	F	F	F	O

Syndrome	CLP	NE	LI	A	C	R	V	CHL	SNL
Oral-facial-digital (OFD I)				P	F	O		I	
Osteochondromuscular dystrophy						P	F	P	
Osteogenesis imperfecta								F	F
Otopalatodigital syndrome	F			F	F	F		F	
Palatopharyngeal incompetence				F		F			
Pendred hypothyroidism, deafness									F
Pfeiffer acroecephalosyndactyly, broad thumb and hallux				F	O	O		F	
Photomyoclonus, diabetes, deafness, cerebral dysfunction		F							F
Prader-Willi syndrome hypotonia, hypogenitalism			F	F	F	O			
Progeroid short stature, pigmented nevi		F					F		F
Pterygium, multiple	F							F	
Pterygium, popliteal	F			F		F		F	
Pyknodysostosis				F					
Refsum hereditary motor and sensory neuropathy		F							F
Robinow fetal face, short forearms, hypoplastic genitalia	F			F		F		F	
Rubella embryopathy			F	F	F				F
Rubenstein-Taybi broad thumbs, beaked nose, slanted eyes				F	F	F		P	
Saethre-Chotzen maxillary hypoplasia, syndactyly				O	O	O		P	
Seckel short stature, prominent nose			F	P	F			P	
Short stature, hyperextensibility, hernia (SHORT)		F	F					F	
Shprintzen-Goldberg craniosynostosis, arachnodactyly				F	F		F		
Sickle cell anemia									F
Simosa elongated craniofacial syndrome				F		F			
Simpson dysmorphia bulldog face, clumsiness, tethered tongue				F			F		
Smith-Magenis brachycephaly, speech and voice disorder		F	F				F		F

Table 3.5 (continued)

Syndrome	CLP	NE	LI	A	C	R	V	CHL	SNL
Sotos cerebral gigantism				F	F				
Speech development delayed, face asymmetry, strabismus				F					
Spondyloepiphyseal dysplasia	F			F	O	F		F	F
Spondylometaphyseal dysplasia, X-linked		F	F		F				
Stickler flat face, myopia, spondyloepi-physeal dysplasia	F			F		F		F	F
Storage-glutamyl-5-phosphate[d]			F	F	F		F	F	F
Storage-lysosomal IVB adult (gangliosidosis GM$_1$)[d]				O	I			F	F
Storage-lysosomal: gangliosidosis, GM$_2$, A(M)B[d]			F	F	F		F	F	F
Storage-lysosomal: Hunter[d]			F	F	F		F	F	F
Storage-lysosomal: Hurler[d]			F	F	F		F	F	F
Storage-lysosomal: Leroy[d]				F	F		F	F	P
Storage-lysosomal: Mannosidosis alpha B[d]			F	F	F		F	F	F
Storage-lysosomal: Mannosidosis B[d]			F	F	F		F	F	F
Storage-lysosomal: Maroteaux-Lamy[d]				F			O	F	P
Storage-lysosomal: Morquio[d]					O		F	F	P
Storage-lysosomal: Pseudo-Hurler[d]				P	F		P	P	P
Storage-lysosomal: Sanfilippo[d]			F	F	F		P	F	P
Storage-lysosomal: Scheie[d]				O	I			F	F
Storage-lysosomal: Schilder (α-galactosidase B)[d]		F	F						
Storage-sialic acid[d]		F	F						
Syndactyly I, microcephaly, mental retardation		F	F						
Treacher-Collins mandibulofacial dysostosis	F			F	O	F		F	O
Usher retinitis pigmentosa, deafness					O				F
Van der Woude lip pit/cleft lip	F			F		F		F	

Syndrome	CLP	NE	LI	A	C	R	V	CHL	SNL
Velocardiofacial syndrome (Shprintzen)	F			F	F	F		F	I
Waardenburg central albinism, hypertelorism, deafness	O			O		O		O	
Weaver macrocephaly, small nose, camptodactyly	O			F	F	O		O	
Williams patulous lips, voice defect, heart malformation				F	F		F		
Wilson hepatolenticular degeneration		F		F	F				

CLP = cleft lip/palate; NE = neurologic abnormalities; LI = learning impairment; A = articulation impairment; C = cognitive impairment; R = resonance impairment; V = voice impairment; CHL = conductive hearing loss; SNL = sensorineural hearing loss; F = frequent; I = infrequent; O = occasional; P = probable. If there is no code in a column, it means that a speech and language problem is part of the syndrome but it could not be determined from the data in the literature if the impairment coded in that column was present or absent.
[a] Characteristics of chromosome disorders include various multiple congenital anomalies and mental deficiency.
[b] Representative of X-linked syndromes of mental retardation with similar speech and language disorders.
[c] Representative of recessive syndromes of mental retardation with similar speech and language disorders.
[d] Characteristics of storage disorders include coarsening features and deterioration of cognition and health.
Sources: Adapted from VA McKusick. Mendelian Inheritance in Man. Catalogues of Autosomal Dominant, Autosomal Recessive, and X-linked Phenotypes (10th ed). Baltimore: Johns Hopkins Press, 1992; KL Jones. Smith's Recognizable Patterns of Human Malformation (4th ed) Philadelphia: Saunders, 1988; and V Siegel-Sadewitz, RJ Shprintzen. The relationship of communication disorders to syndrome identification. J Speech Hearing Disord 1982;47:338.

REFERENCES

1. Thurmon TF. Mutagens, Radiation, and Teratogens: Modern Witches. Shreveport, LA: Grand Rounds, LSU Medical Center, 1991.
2. McKusick VA. Mendelian Inheritance in Man. Catalogues of Autosomal Dominant, Autosomal Recessive, and X-Linked Phenotypes (10th ed). Baltimore: Johns Hopkins Press, 1992;251.
3. Sever JL, Ellenberg JH, Ley AC, et al. Toxoplasmosis: maternal and pediatric findings in 23,000 pregnancies. Pediatrics 1988;82:181.
4. Thurmon TF. Medical Genetics Primer. Shreveport, LA: LSUMC-S Bookstore, 1997.
5. Carter CO. Multifactorial Genetic Disease. In VA McKusick, R Claiborne (eds), Medical Genetics. New York: Hospital Practice Publishers, 1973.
6. Locke JL, Mather PL. Genetic factors in the ontogeny of spoken language: evidence from monozygotic and dizygotic twins. J Child Lang 1989;16:553.
7. Gilger JW. Genetics in disorders of language. Clin Commun Disord 1992;2:35.
8. Van Camp G, Willems PJ, Smith RJH. Nonsyndromic hearing impairment: unparalleled heterogeneity. Am J Hum Genet 1997;60:758.
9. Dykens E. Psychologists and geneticists: two cultures. Am J Hum Genet 1996;59:29.

4

The Early Intervention Team: Giving and Getting the Right Kind of Help

Frances P. Billeaud

Whether services are provided to infants, toddlers, and their families under the traditional clinical model or under the Part H/Part C Early Intervention Model, speech-language pathologists (SLPs) are clearly members of a team effort. The team manager, or captain, is always the person or persons with the ultimate decision-making authority, that is, the parents. The reality of parents as team managers has always been true, but professionals have sometimes conceptualized themselves as the true leaders, possibly because parents invest the professionals they have chosen with significant authority in the initial stages of the team relationship. During that early period, families are faced with making difficult decisions about their child's care that they never dreamed would be required of them. Simultaneously, they are coping as best they can with the emotional and financial implications for their family's future after having received the news, or confirmation of their suspicion, that their child is in need of specialized care.

Early intervention teams can have many members who represent several professional specialties or can be made up of the parents and one or two professionals, depending on the needs of the child and his or her family. Team functioning is possible across all professional settings; however, making the transition from the traditional clinical operational philosophy, which relies on the collective knowledge and skills contributed by independent practitioners, to one that relies on effective parent-professional partnerships requires a high level of trust among the team members, commitment to implementation of the best practices, willingness to exert the effort, and leadership. Change is never easy, and systems change is extremely difficult, but it is both possible and desirable if undertaken for the right reasons.

Luterman[1] observed that "[p]arents and professionals in speech-language pathology are natural allies. They both want in the most ardent terms the same thing: a child with better communicating skills" (p. 175).

FAMILY AS FOCUS OF THE TEAM EFFORT

The family chooses members of the intervention or treatment team for the primary purpose of getting help for their child. At the outset, they may see the selection of professionals as their only contribution to that end, expecting the professionals they have selected to "fix" or "cure" the problem. As their understanding of the nature of communicative delays and disorders evolves, and it becomes clear that day-to-day activities within the family are part of effective treatment, their roles as team members become more diverse. Under the Individuals with Disabilities Education Act (IDEA) model, in fact, a goal of intervention is to empower the family itself to enhance the child's development. Thus, professionals working with infants and toddlers with communicative delays and disorders spend significant amounts of time planning interventions together with the parents; receiving information about the child's activities and behaviors in the home setting, family routines, and cultural and child-rearing practices; and engaging in ongoing evaluation of the effectiveness of intervention and therapy strategies applied in the home setting. Practitioners provide parental guidance, parent education, parent training, and counseling, all as part of the management package.

Thus, families who contact professionals for assistance come with varying levels of information about their child's condition, which is the reason they are seeking help. On some level (they know it, they suspect it, they were told it), there is knowledge that "something is not right." They expect the professional or team of professionals to offer help. They may have a particular kind of help in mind or may entrust the decision about what kind of help is appropriate to the professionals. Just as they have the right to select the professionals on their team, they have the right to add others to the team, terminate services, resume services after a hiatus, seek second opinions, and change service providers. Families have always had such options, but professionals who were trained to believe that their own protocols took precedence over family choices have often judged the exercise of the options as evidence of noncompliance on the part of families. A decade of experience with the Part H approach has modified the thinking of the professional community to some extent, but the advent of managed care may shape philosophies of best practices in a somewhat different direction.

Family Systems Theory in Practice

It is obvious that parent-professional teams are essential in optimizing treatment, management, and intervention outcomes. Practitioners find it useful to consider the family unit from the perspective of family systems theory, because an understanding of the individual child's family helps to formulate effective treatment plans that require family participation. Systems theory can be helpful when thinking about how families operate as they do. Summers and colleagues[2] and Wayman and colleagues[3] suggested that the family system can be considered as interrelationships among the following:

- Family structure: the number of people in the family, their respective relationships to each other, and their values and beliefs
- Family interaction: the manner in which the individual members interact with the others and their places or roles within the family unit
- Family functions: the responsibilities the family unit bears to its members
- Family life cycle: those alterations in family structure, function, and interaction that occur over time in the course of daily living

A family is sensitive to the ebb and flow of many events, stresses, pleasures, and challenges that affect both individual members and the collective unit. Professionals must be sensitive both to family members with whom there is direct or indirect interaction and to the stresses, issues, and values that they recognize as influencing their lives and family functioning.

As Luterman[1] pointed out, families of handicapped children are not necessarily dysfunctional families (although some may be), but they are families that are under stress. The presence of a child with special needs affects different families in different ways. It strengthens family bonds for some and, perhaps, places unbearable stress on families that are already fragile. Professionals who provide services to youngsters who have or are at risk for disabilities involving communicative disorders encounter a broad spectrum of coping abilities and responses among the families.

Parents who have looked back on the time at which they first suspected or learned for certain that their child had a significant problem have reported feelings that range from shock and confusion to anger and despair. Some have reported moving through stages of grief much like those that Kubler-Ross[4] described in relation to experiencing a terminal illness or the death of a loved one. On the other hand, some parents reported being readily accepting of the news, especially if there were other family members affected by the same condition.[5,6]

The personal experience of one family illustrates the importance of being sensitive to the emotional plight of the parents:

When we as parents come to the professionals, begging for services . . . there is another angry little voice inside us that says, "Why does this have to be?" This angry little voice is loud. Behind the anger is fear, big time fear. Fear of the unknown, fear of losing something precious, fear of failure.

My child was diagnosed . . . with a severe language disorder. For well over a year after he was diagnosed, I was devastated. My reaction was completely disproportionate to the reality. . . . It was very hard for me. I had to deal with it on a daily basis. I'm the one who watched as some moms went to the park while we went to therapy. My instinct to protect my child couldn't slow down the ever-widening gap between my child and his friends.

My nightmare was that I would be judged to be unfit and he would be taken away (my nightmare stems from the fact that my older sister who is severely mentally retarded and an epileptic was taken away when I was four).

As I said, not terribly rational, but this is what we [parents] are dealing with. A parent in this state is just trying to defuse the sense of failure, powerlessness, and anger. Even if the service is desperately needed and the parent accepts it, the underlying loss of parental power and self-esteem is there.[7]

Sometimes the presentation of a diagnosis of a significant developmental problem is as hard for the professional to make as it is for the family to hear. Consideration for the feelings of the family as they receive diagnostic information and recommendations about follow-up management should be a concern of professionals whose role it is to interact with families about those matters. Because diagnosis and assessment are often the family's first encounters with labels their child may have, it is also important for the professional to present information to the family about what the diagnostic label implies with respect to eligibility for treatment and management programs, selection of appropriate intervention strategies, and their right to confidentiality of records relating to their child. The amount of information that can be absorbed by a family at one time is limited, especially at a time when diagnosis of a significant disability is presented. Gauging how much information to provide at that time is another responsibility of the practitioner.

Some families may be in crisis when they are first encountered. For example, their child may be suffering from a serious illness or recovering from surgical or medical treatments required to preserve the child's life. They may be preoccupied with financial or logistical problems that require their full energies and resources. Until the crisis is resolved, it will probably be difficult, if not impossible, for family members to participate constructively in the management of their child's needs, beyond the provision of basic care. Sometimes even that contribution is beyond the family's ability. In such cases, social welfare agencies or the courts may find it necessary to remove the child from the family for a period of time, so that the primary caregivers can receive appropriate assistance for themselves.

If the family is viewed from the systems perspective, then the child's environment can be considered ecologically. Again, everything within the family environment affects every member of the family in some way to a greater or lesser extent. This concept is useful both from a philosophical point of view and in practical applications of interventions. Because the concept is likely to be a new one to family members themselves, it may be helpful to introduce it early during the formation of the parent-professional team. The family-needs assessment, required under Part H/Part C regulations, can begin with an eco-mapping process that assists the family to recognize its specific strengths (resources); needs (areas of concern); and the interrelationships among activities, agencies, and family functions. The process of eco-mapping is an efficient and practical strategy to help the family select and prioritize the services they desire.

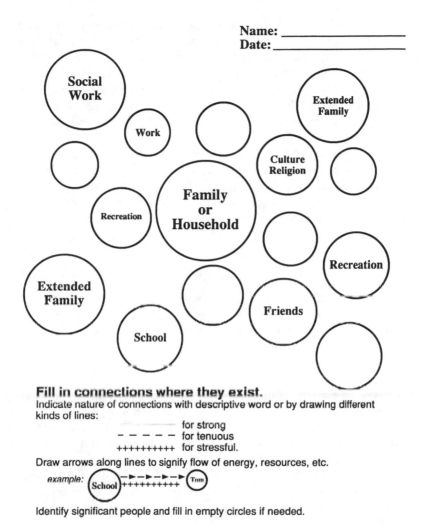

Figure 4.1 Eco-map. (Reprinted with permission of The Free Press, a division of Macmillan, Inc., from *Family-Centered Social Work Practice* by Ann Hartman and Joan Laird. © 1983 by The Free Press.)

The Eco-Map

Hartman and Laird[8] provided a format for developing the eco-map (Figure 4.1). The family identifies its members (their names are written in the center circle). Connections between the family and its associations and activities (shown in the other circles) are indicated by different kinds of lines. Heavy, bold lines represent strong, positive connections; narrower solid lines indicate ongoing positive or neutral connections; railroad-like lines highlight stressful connections; dotted lines indicate tenuous relationships or other important connections that the family feels unable to assess accurately. Arrows signify the flow of energy, resources, and effort toward or away from the family unit. The resulting picture—the eco-map—becomes a tool created by the family, which can be used as a basis for discussing prospective family resources and areas of concern or need. This insight can be useful in planning and shaping components of the intervention program. The eco-map can be modified as conditions within and around the family change.

After development of the eco-map, other tools used in the family-needs assessment can then be selected and interpreted in light of knowledge of a particular family system. Questionnaires can be used to identify areas of personal and social resources, service coordination, and time management. Information provided through such tools is more meaningful when considered in light of the family system.

Family Configurations, Demographics, and Cultural Considerations

Families are different in today's world than they were even in the fairly recent past. The demographics of our society speak for themselves. One of six children lives in a single-parent home. One of every two black children lives in a single-parent home headed by a woman. In 1986, almost three-fourths of all black infants were born to unwed mothers; half of the mothers were teenagers. Increasing numbers of preterm, very-low-birth-weight, sick infants are being born to women who have had inadequate (or no) prenatal care; most of those babies are being saved by advanced medical technology. Many survive with impairments, and their families require a range of resources. By the year 2000, 38% of all children under the age of 18 will be from minority families. The fastest growing segment of the country's population is Asian American. Hispanic Americans also represent an expanding portion of the population; in some areas of the country Hispanic Americans already constitute the majority of residents. In contrast, the professional community continues to be underrepresented by practitioners from minority groups.[9]

Clearly, services provided to many segments of the population are influenced by cultural practices and languages that differ from those of the majority of the professional community. Further, the family's cultural perspectives regarding child-rearing practices and interactions with health care providers and educators, handicapping conditions, and appropriate intervention or management strategies can differ significantly from those of the practitioners seeking to provide a child with beneficial services. The practitioner must seek to understand and appreciate the cultural variety of society and be sensitive to the issues that can bring the traditionally trained professional and the family into potential conflict.[10]

Participants at the 1989 conference discussing services to infants and children from culturally diverse backgrounds, conducted by the National Center for Clinical Infant Programs, identified a number of issues of importance to practitioners who serve young children. The conference report[11] is a useful resource for professionals who seek to enhance their knowledge of cultural perceptions and practices. The authors remind us that there are cultural and situational influences that, if ignored, can doom to failure from the outset even the best-intentioned programs for handicapped and at-risk infants and toddlers.

Among the cultural issues that must be considered are (1) how people feel about, manifest, and treat the states of health and illness and physical, mental, and emotional disabilities; (2) the group of people who are considered to be family members and the relationships these people have to one another; (3) child-rearing techniques; and, (4) in addition to the language of the home, the various ways in which people communicate. It is important to remember that situational and environmental conditions such as poverty, homelessness, lack of formal education, and other factors that put children and families at grave risk are *not* cultural attributes but are variables that cut across all cultures.

This overview of some of the issues that affect the practitioner's relationship with families from culturally diverse backgrounds is included because of the ecologic importance of cultural influences. Competent pediatric practitioners recognize the necessity of being sensitive to potential barriers and possible means of avoiding them in the course of providing services to children with special needs whose family cultures differ from their own.

It is possible to develop sensitivity to the factors that are important in working with a given family. Wayman and colleagues[3] developed a useful set of guidelines for early interventionists who have responsibility for home visits. Their approach suggests that it is important to understand family structure, customary patterns of caregiving, child-rearing practices, family schedules, and family responses to the child's behaviors. The family's attitude and perceptions about the child's disability, health, and health care are also important, as are the family's language use (is an interpreter needed?) and interactional styles (is there a designated family spokesperson or leader?). Wayman and colleagues guide practitioners into productive areas of inquiry and observation under each of these areas. The guidelines are equally valuable to practitioners who work with families in settings other than the home. The site of service provision does not diminish the need to understand and respect the family within which the child lives.

Expectations

The expectations of the family and the professional constitute another set of issues about which sensitivity needs to be developed. Luterman[1] emphasized the importance of each party's understanding of the other's expectations of what is to occur during assessment and treatment programs, what each expects the other to contribute, and the outcomes that each expect. Failure to understand the expectations vested in the process and the people involved is often the root of failure to achieve a successful, collaborative team effort for the benefit of the child with special needs.

Parents should be provided with information about the practitioner's expectations as the stages of their association advance. For example, it may be helpful to provide the family with information sheets that outline the typical process and sequence of events involved in evaluation and assessment activities. Such information not only prepares them for the unfamiliar series of events, but can also help them organize their questions, ideas, and observations, thus enhancing their ability to participate effectively.

Likewise, the professional should seek to discover the family's expectations. This can be done through a number of techniques, but the most successful is probably a face-to-face discussion, which validates the practitioner's interest in the family's concerns and has the advantage of immediacy.

Parents can be active partners in all phases of the assessment and intervention process, not merely signers of informed consents or requests-for-service forms (unless that is the role they choose to play). When this philosophy of parents as active partners is applied, the assessment process itself can become the first step in intervention or treatment. The concept is not a new one, but the means of implementing collaborative parent-professional partnerships can present challenges for which most communication disorders professionals have not been formally trained.

Table 4.1 summarizes some of the means through which a collaborative parent-professional partnership can emerge.

Blosser (p. 34)[12] summarized the contributions families make to the SLP's development of management plans appropriate to their particular situation as follows:

- The American family is diverse. *Consider each family's unique state of being when making recommendations and planning treatment.*
- Each person has a unique coping style. *Strive to identify the coping styles demonstrated by your client's family members and select counseling and education techniques accordingly.*
- Family members know their loved one better than you. They have much to contribute to the assessment, planning, and intervention process. *Develop strategies for incorporating family into every phase of treatment.*
- Technology offers clinicians opportunities to reach family members when they might otherwise be inaccessible. *Be familiar with technological resources; expand your resource library.*
- Families come in all shapes and sizes and are not defined only by blood relationships. *Identify those individuals who share a special relationship with your client and foster their awareness and skills.*

Under the parent-professional team model, the child with special needs is provided with a management program that involves the entire ecosystem (family and community) in which he or she lives. Those who care most about their child with special needs are directly involved in planning and conducting activities that enhance the child's development.

Table 4.1 Parent-Professional Partnerships: Some Collaborative Activities

Parent and Family Roles	Practitioner Roles
Family assessment of strengths and needs	Selection of tools and approaches (e.g., eco-map, interview, questionnaires)
Identifying priorities for the child concerning communicative development	Eliciting assistance of the family in identifying how the child communicates
	Presenting, clarifying, and exploring treatment options
Acquiring new information about pre-communicative development and emerging communicative skills	Identifying parents' preferred learning methods and providing instruction in an appropriate format
Integrating communicative stimulation into daily routines	Providing information with regard to short-term goals and their connection to targeted priorities
	Showing how play is used as a vehicle for communication
Recording data to track the child's communicative status and development	Training in data-keeping skills Selecting appropriate formats
Stimulating, teaching, and modeling language and speech	Modeling, demonstrating, and teaching specific communicative skills
	Coaching, validating efforts, and affirming skills
Accepting and using power to influence child's continuing development	All of the roles listed above
	Talking with (not to or at) the family
Collaborating in evaluation of outcomes and options in ongoing intervention activities	Counseling
	Selecting or providing the forum and means of documentation
Accepting transitions as they become appropriate	Preparing family for service, setting, personnel, program, priority, and relationship changes
Helping the professional to accept transitions as they become appropriate	

SPEECH-LANGUAGE PATHOLOGISTS AS MULTIDISCIPLINARY TEAM MEMBERS

SLPs and audiologists who serve infants, toddlers, and their families must be able to work with very young children whose needs vary widely; whose histories, diagnoses, etiologies, and prognoses differ significantly; and whose families' needs for guidance are equally diverse. It should be obvious that communicative disorders specialists often work together with specialists from many other disciplines to meet the needs of affected children and their families. Sometimes, however, the team is composed of the communicative disorders specialist and the family with only occasional contacts with other professionals. Although children who are identified as "at risk" on or shortly following birth are probably under the care of medical specialists, other professionals may be the first to recognize the need for intervention services, especially among children whose condition is recognized after the first birthday.

Multidisciplinary evaluation and assessment are required to establish eligibility and initiate intervention under federal Part H/Part C regulations and companion state statutes. Federal regulations stipulate that at least two professional disciplines be involved in evaluation and assessment activities and allow participation by as many professional disciplines as is necessary to complete a thorough assessment and develop an appropriate Individual Family Services Plan (IFSP).

Knowledge, Skills, and Competencies Expected of the Speech-Language Pathologist

The SLP who serves infants and toddlers diagnosed with or at risk for delays, disorders, and disabilities and their families in any setting must have considerable knowledge in a variety of areas. This knowledge must supplement the basic general knowledge acquired by every SLP about communicative development and disorders of communication.

Knowledge

Specifically, SLPs who work with this population must have in-depth information about the following:

- Prenatal development and potential problems associated with the prenatal environment, teratogens, genetic considerations, and maternal health during pregnancy
- Developmental anatomy, physiology, neurologic sequences, and the implications of problems that are associated with each area
- Normal infant development across all areas (i.e., physical, neuromotor, social, emotional, and cognitive)
- Sequelae of specific diagnosed conditions with regard to communicative development and the early development that precedes symbolic communication
- Family systems
- Roles, functions, and skills of other professional disciplines that are involved with the care of infants, toddlers, and their families
- Customary treatments and technologies used by related professionals in their work with young children at risk for or diagnosed with delays or disabilities
- Referral criteria and protocols used to secure consultations when there are suspected problems or there is need for specific information
- Pertinent laws, regulations, entitlements, and programs that are available to the population, and the eligibility requirements for each
- How to access services in the community that may be needed by families of affected children and by the children themselves
- Effective interviewing methods, techniques, and options

- Terminology used by other disciplines so that the professional can (1) understand their reports, (2) be able to interpret information to the family accurately, and (3) communicate with professional colleagues
- The limits of personal and professional practice, referring to other service providers as their expertise is required or appropriate
- How to handle and position infants who require specialized care
- How to conduct feeding and swallowing assessments and perform interventions with infants who exhibit problems in those areas
- The options for multidisciplinary team composition and functioning in various settings

Skills and Competencies

Skills and competencies that the SLP must be able to demonstrate in working with this population likewise are specialized. They represent skills and competencies over and above those the SLP is expected to possess in working with older communicatively impaired individuals and include the following:

- Participating effectively as a multidisciplinary team member
- Conducting screenings to identify atypical communicative development (including presymbolic communicative development and nonverbal forms of communicative development)
- Contributing accurate and clearly worded information to other professionals who work with the child and family and to family members
- Conducting assessments of current levels of communicative development for purposes of developing appropriate treatment, management, or intervention plans
- Exercising effective listening skills with family members and other service providers
- Conducting family interviews to obtain case-history information
- Providing effective family counseling concerning communicative development, referrals, legal rights, community services, and other matters within the scope of professional practice
- Conducting communicative diagnoses separate from or as a part of a larger diagnostic effort
- Conducting examination of the oral mechanism
- Assessing respiratory effort in vocalization
- Assessing receptive communication and expressive communication (including presymbolic and symbolic stages, vocal, verbal, and nonverbal)
- Integrating data supplied by the audiologist and others with regard to its effect on the child's communicative development
- Conducting family-needs assessments (as related to the family's desire and ability to enhance the child's development)
- Participating in planning appropriate management for communication delays and disorders (per IFSP or other care-plan requirements as appropriate)

- Participating in conducting appropriate management programs, both direct and indirect, and combinations of direct and indirect strategies
- Evaluating outcomes of management programs
- Referring children and their families to appropriate services as needed (e.g., medical: pediatricians, neurologists, ophthalmologists, orthopedists, otorhinolaryngologists, allergists, plastic surgeons, oral surgeons, geneticists, early and periodic screening, diagnosis, and treatment clinics, handicapped children's health services, and allied health services such as occupational and physical therapy; dental; nutrition; social services: financial assistance, transportation, support groups, daycare, respite care; psychological; and developmental services)
- Interacting with other service providers who conduct portions of the child's total developmental program (e.g., infant interventionists, assessment teachers, noncategorical preschool handicapped teachers, daycare providers, social workers, physical therapists, occupational therapists, adapted physical education personnel)
- Collaborating on service provision activities where and when possible (i.e., planning, conducting, and evaluating outcomes)
- Coordinating some or all of the services needed by the child (i.e., family service coordination, formerly designated *case-management services*)
- Planning transitions with the multidisciplinary team, including the family
- Planning transitions before their occurrence

It is clear that the professional competencies needed by the practitioner do not rest on simple downward extensions of knowledge and skills appropriate to the mature child or adult.[13]

Role of the Speech-Language Pathologist

The SLP practitioner can serve in many roles within and across service-delivery settings. At various times, the SLP serves as a source of information, parent trainer, parent educator, family support professional, SLP, diagnostician, researcher, team participant, service coordinator, advisor, counselor, promoter of public awareness, advocate for the child and for early intervention programs, and professional educator. Throughout these activities, the practitioner also remains an individual, who must acknowledge and deal with personal sensitivities, vulnerabilities, biases, values, and the need to continue learning and growing professionally.[1]

It is important that the SLP's roles be recognized by other team members and by family members. Unfortunately, the general public and service providers in other disciplines are often uninformed about the various roles performed by SLPs and audiologists for the target population. Indeed, professionals in related disciplines tend to be underinformed about communicative development in general—an issue that is also of concern to SLPs who serve the infant-toddler population (and an issue that presents ongoing opportunities for offering continuing-education programs designed for professionals as well as family members). There is much work to be done in the area of public awareness and marketing the services of communicative disorders specialists. Chapter 10 addresses this subject.

Speech-language pathology services for the infant/toddler population include several broad categories, within which are clusters of more specific services. The broad service categories are

- Prevention services
- Diagnosis and assessment services
- Planning of treatment and intervention programs
- Implementation of treatment and intervention programs
- Professional consultation and referral services
- Resource-coordination services (service coordination)
- Parent-training services (individualized to specific needs)
- Parent-education services (group and individual)
- Counseling services
- Transition planning and implementation services

Depending on the type and setting of the SLP's professional practice, services can be offered on a one-time only basis (e.g., consultation with attending professionals and referral of families to speech-language services or developmental programs nearer their homes), on an intensive short-term basis (e.g., providing services during the infant's stay in the neonatal intensive care unit or intermediate-care nursery before discharge or providing short-term intervention to facilitate language development in late talkers), or on an intermittent basis (e.g., assessment services provided in follow-up clinics when the goal is training, ongoing therapeutic, and other services to an infant with a diagnosed condition that entails atypical communicative development).

The argument, if there is to be one, is not whether SLPs should be prepared to deliver services in one manner or another, or one setting or another, but rather how the needs of the children and families who seek services can be met effectively in any setting.

The Speech-Language Pathologist and Community Settings

SLPs can be used in a number of settings that bring them in contact with professionals from other disciplines and with at-risk or disabled infants, toddlers, and their families. The SLP is expected to bring to the team specialized knowledge of communicative development and of factors that can interfere with that development or modify its form, the ability to assess capabilities and limitations or barriers involving a particular child and family, and the ability to work with other members of the team to plan and execute appropriate strategies to optimize the child's development.

The settings in which practitioners function influence the array of services provided and their focus. For example, services provided in a neonatal intensive care unit differ from those provided in the home, daycare center, or developmental services program. Whatever the setting, it is essential to remember that SLPs and audiologists who work with infants, toddlers, and families are never solo practitioners. They are always part of a team. The minimum team for the communicatively impaired child is composed of the parent(s), the child, providers of the child's health care, and the communicative disorders specialist. The team often has other members as well (e.g., other family members, daycare providers, early childhood special educators, psychologists).

SUMMARY

The idea of team functioning is not new in itself, but the importance of thinking of ourselves as team members has recently received renewed emphasis and validation in light of the mandates imposed under IDEA.[14-20] Ultimately, the team is "quarterbacked" or managed by the parents, who make decisions about their child's care and participate in treatment and management programs to the extent that they choose.

REFERENCES

1. Luterman DM. Counseling the Communicatively Disordered and Their Families (2nd ed). Austin, TX: Pro-Ed, 1991;175.
2. Summers JA, Brotherson MJ, Turnbull AP. The Impact of Handicapped Children on Families. In EW Lynch, RB Lewis (eds), Exceptional Children and Adults. Glenville, IL: Scott-Foresman, 1988;504.
3. Wayman KI, Lynch EW, Hanson MJ. Home-based early childhood services: cultural sensitivity in a family systems approach. Top Early Child Special Educ 1991;10:56.
4. Kubler-Ross E. On Death and Dying. New York: Macmillan, 1969.
5. Billeaud FP. Region IV Interagency Coordinating Council Needs Assessment Report. Lafayette, LA: Region IV Interagency Coordinating Council, 1989.
6. Borland B. Parents' Responses to a Child's Problems. In C Semmler (ed), A Guide to the Care and Management of Very Low Birth Weight Infants. Tucson, AZ: Therapy Skill Builders, 1989;11.
7. Dawkins C. Address to the Louisiana Interagency Coordinating Council. Lafayette, LA, November 1990.
8. Hartman A, Laird J. Family-Centered Social Work Practice. New York: Free Press, 1983.
9. American Speech-Language-Hearing Association. Semiannual Counts of the ASHA Membership and Affiliation for the Period January 1 through June 30, 1996. Rockville, MD: American Speech-Language-Hearing Association, 1996.
10. Lynch EW, Hanson MJ. Developing Cross-Cultural Competence: A Guide for Working with Young Children and Their Families. Baltimore: Paul H. Brookes, 1992.
11. Anderson PP, Fenichel ES. Serving Culturally Diverse Families of Infants and Toddlers with Disabilities. Washington, DC: National Center for Clinical Infant Programs, 1989.
12. Blosser J. Working with families: making time count. ASHA 1996;38:34.
13. Peterson NL, Siegel-Causey E, Copeland ME, Dale DA. Personal Training Competencies for Interventionists Serving Infants with Disabilities and At-Risk Conditions (Birth through Age 2). Lawrence, KS: University of Kansas, 1988.

14. Bailey DB, Simeonsson RS, Huntington GS, et al. Preparing Professionals from Multiple Disciplines to Work with Handicapped Infants, Toddlers and Their Families: Current Status and Future Directions. Paper presented at the International Early Childhood Conference on Children with Special Needs, Nashville, TN, November 1988.
15. Dunst CJ, Trivette C, Deal A. Enabling and Empowering Families, Principles and Guidelines for Practice. Cambridge, MA: Brookline Press, 1988.
16. Sparks SN. Assessing Infants and Toddlers: A Family Focus. ASHA Videoconference, Rockville, MD, May 1989.
17. Sparks SN. Assessment and intervention with at-risk infants and toddlers: guidelines for the speech-language pathologist. Top Lang Disord 1989;10:43.
18. Shonkoff JA. Perspective on Pediatric Training. In J Mulic, S Pueschel (eds), Parent-Professional Partnerships in Developmental Disability Services. Cambridge, MA: Ware Press, 1983;75.
19. Shonkoff J, Hauser-Cram P. Early intervention for disabled infants and their families: a quantitative analysis. Pediatrics 1987;80:650.
20. Shonkoff J, Hauser-Cram P, Krauss MW, Upshaw C. Early intervention efficacy research—what have we learned and where do we go from here? Top Early Child Special Educ 1988;8:81.

5

Role of the Speech-Language Pathologist in the Neonatal Intensive Care Unit: Preemies, Micropreemies, and Medically Fragile Infants

Frances P. Billeaud

The speech-language pathologist (SLP) whose practice includes work in the neonatal intensive care unit (NICU) provides a number of services, each of which requires specialized preparation. Roles can include services provided to and for NICU staff, parents, and families of the infants, as well as direct services to the infants themselves.[1] Services can focus solely on communicative interactions or include consultation and parent education and training in regard to the oral feeding and other oral motor activities from which the coordinated movements required for speech development evolve.[2,3]

Before detailing the functions of the SLP in executing such specialized roles, it may be helpful to consider the hospital setting in which the services are rendered. The NICU is only one of several units that compose the hospital complex. As a part of the hospital, the NICU must adhere to established standards in terms of physical space, equipment, staff, procedural protocols, and provision of patient care. General requirements for NICUs are prescribed by the Joint Commission on Hospital Accreditation, and maintenance of accreditation is dependent on ongoing compliance with those requirements.

Once a baby leaves the delivery room, the legal responsibility for care rests with the designated attending physician(s). Depending on hospital policy, the NICU level, the child's needs, and the family's wishes, the physician may be a family practitioner, a pediatrician, a neonatologist, a pediatric subspecialist (e.g., pediatric gastroenterologist, pediatric cardiologist, pediatric neurosurgeon), or a team of specialists. Because of legal and ethical responsibilities, other professionals are called in by the attending physician(s) to provide specific services. No services are provided without orders from the attending physician(s).

If the infant is admitted to the NICU, many professionals participate in caring for the child. Staffing patterns in the NICU usually place one nurse on each shift in charge of from one to four infants. Nurses are responsible for executing the nursing care plan for their assigned infant(s). Other staff typically found in the NICU include neonatologists, occupational and physical therapists, case managers, SLPs, social workers, pastoral care providers, dietitians and nutritionists, clinical nurse specialists, and utilization review personnel, all of whom function as part of the multidisciplinary team. The staff also includes technicians who operate specialized equipment (e.g., x-ray and brain-scanning equipment to detect anomalies and intracranial hemorrhages), housekeeping staff who keep floors and other surfaces clean, and maintenance personnel. Parents are also in and out of the unit on a regular basis. Administrative staff make their rounds in the unit on a regular basis. The hub of all the activity, of course, is the infant population, most of whom are connected to a variety of monitors. Lights flash, monitor screens glow with the changing configurations of electronic traces, monitors and alarms hum and buzz to indicate the status of infants' various bodily functions. Beepers page personnel, telephones ring, and incoming and outgoing calls are placed or answered. The NICU is a busy place!

In keeping with hospital policy, detailed charting is maintained of all services provided while the infant is in the facility. Patient records are subject to review by various staff members and hospital committees designated by the hospital (e.g., quality assurance, institutional review board, infant mortality, infection control, medical ethics) and by representatives of their accreditation bodies. Medical records are also subject to subpoena by the judicial system when disputes arise about legal issues. One of the professional's most important responsibilities is to maintain accurate records in a timely manner.

NEWBORN CARE OPTIONS: NEONATAL INTENSIVE CARE VERSUS OTHER SETTINGS

Many levels of newborn care are available to modern medicine, including at least three levels of intensive care. The condition of the infant at birth generally dictates where neonatal care is provided. There are at least four choices in the hospital system, each level having an increasingly sophisticated capability for dealing with the infant's needs.

Rooming-In Care

Rooming-in allows the mother and her healthy baby to be in the same room throughout the hospital stay, with medical and nursing staff nearby to provide support and care as needed. Rooming-in, with its liberal visiting privileges, provides a home-like environment for the family, while maintaining ready access to medical treatment. Under this option, hospital stay for mother and child is usually brief, usually only a day or two.

Level I Nursery Care (Well-Baby Nursery)

Admission to the level I nursery is probably the most common form of newborn care provided in this country. The nursing staff cares for the babies in a common nursery area, which grandparents and friends can view through plate-glass windows. Trips out of the nursery are limited to visiting the mother's room for bottle or breast feedings or periods of nurturing and cuddling. Following delivery, healthy infants and their mothers are usually discharged after a stay of 12–24 hours after vaginal delivery and 72 hours after cesarean section delivery (in contrast to the 5- to 7-day confinements common in years past). Treatment for minor problems the infant may develop (e.g., mild jaundice, minor feeding problems) is normally provided in a level I nursery.

Level II and Level III Nursery Care

The level II nursery provides the first level of neonatal intensive care. Level II nurseries were initially designed to serve the needs of preterm infants, or preemies. Their mission has been expanded to include treatment of other infants who require more attention than is usually available in level I nurseries. The level II NICU is staffed by physicians, nurses, allied health personnel, and technicians with specific skills. Highly sophisticated monitoring equipment is at hand to make certain that infants receive adequate oxygenation and nutrition, maintain adequate body temperature, and are treated promptly for any problem. Isolettes, warming tables, phototherapy lights to treat jaundice, equipment to scan for intraventricular hemorrhages, suctions, feeding tubes, and a wide variety of other equipment are available to provide immediate response to each infant's needs. Babies who require monitoring or treatment for a specific problem may spend only a brief time in the level II NICU, before being discharged or returned to the level I unit. Infants who are significantly preterm or who exhibit problems requiring technological support or extended medical treatment may spend several weeks or even months on the unit. Premature babies are not only smaller than babies born at term, but they also have immature neurologic development, which affects their ability to adjust to life outside the womb (respiration, maintenance of body temperature, regulation of biological state, sleep and wake cycles, and sucking and swallowing). The treatment required to help these fragile infants sustain life sometimes places additional stress on their systems and results in short- or long-term problems, for which additional intervention is required once the medical condition has stabilized.

Level III nurseries provide even more sophisticated care for newborns. Level III NICUs are available in fewer hospitals because of the high costs of maintaining the service (which include the cost of high-tech equipment and lower staff-to-patient ratios) and the high level of specialized personnel training required to care for very small, very fragile infants. Although level III units are often located in teaching hospitals, it is becoming increasingly common for hospitals to combine level II and III units within a single physical space, allowing babies to move back and forth between levels of care as their needs require. Infants are frequently transported to level III centers from outlying areas for specialized medical or surgical treatment. Families are often unable to be with their infants during their stay in a level III NICU because of its distance from their homes. Consequently, these sick and fragile babies have a very different start in life than their healthier peers.[4]

As soon as the medical crisis is over, and the infant is strong enough to leave the level III NICU, it is customary to transfer the baby to a step-down unit, in which the expenses of providing any needed continuing care are somewhat lower. Babies can remain in the step-down unit—often a level II NICU—as "growers" until they reach a specified weight, attain full-term age, or are otherwise stable enough medically to be released from hospital care.

Level IV Nurseries

The most sophisticated NICUs are rated as level IV NICUs. There are generally only a few of these in each state. Infants with extremely rare or complex conditions that require highly specialized surgical or medical interventions are often transported to level IV centers for such care.

INVOLVEMENT OF THE SPEECH-LANGUAGE PATHOLOGIST IN NEWBORN CARE

The purpose of all hospitals is to provide treatment for medical and surgical problems presented by their patients, whatever the age, within the role and scope of the institution's mission. The SLP may provide services to children on the pediatric service(s), including the NICU, of a given hospital; provide services across many services (e.g., rehabilitation, out-patient clinics, acute care, pediatrics); or serve only in the NICU, depending on the hospital's structure, mission, administrative philosophy, and staffing patterns. The SLP can serve as a consulting professional, a part-time staff member, or a permanent member of the house staff.

NICU services have developed rapidly as advances in biomedical technology and reliable data on developmental outcomes of an array of management protocols have emerged. The concept of comprehensive neonatal patient care has come to include not only medical treatment but also provision of information, training, and education for family members who now participate in decision making for their infant patients and who are best equipped to provide certain aspects of their care. Other things being equal, infants who are visited regularly by their parents in the NICU tend to do better than those whose families are unable to participate in their care during NICU hospitalization. The primary caregiver's (usually mother's) engagement of the infant through mutual gazing, verbal comforting, early social turn taking, cuddling and stroking, feeding, and rocking all seem to contribute to the baby's biological development and neurobehavioral organization and development.[5-8] (Also see the works of T. Berry Brazelton, Heidelese Als, Forrest Bennett, Gretchen Lawhon, and Craig Ramey for specific references in this regard.)

Involvement in the Level III and Level IV Neonatal Intensive Care Unit

Because babies in the level III and IV NICU are likely to have urgent medical needs that temporarily take priority over their developmental needs, the SLP is less likely to be involved in direct care provision to the baby. However, the SLP may be a regular participant in multidisciplinary team rounds and contribute to the team's ongoing needs assessment and discharge-planning processes.

A consultative role is likely with babies who have a cleft palate and special feeding needs, especially if they are also preterm, small for gestational age, or have a syndrome of which a palatal cleft is one of several features. For example, infants who have poor tongue control often have significantly improved oral feeding ability when a specialized feeder (i.e., Haberman feeder or specially designed nipple) is used or when the tip of the tongue is sutured to the lower lip, which effectively holds it forward in the mouth and away from the airway (the tack is released as the child gains better oral-motor control). The "tacking" procedure also seems to alleviate episodes of breathing problems associated with the tongue's obstruction of the airway. As a rule, whether or not the tongue has been tacked, these babies should be held in a nearly upright position for oral feedings to facilitate gravitational assistance in fluid intake.

Families are encouraged to visit and gradually participate in the care of their infants in the level III and IV settings. In the initial stages, they too may be limited to bedside visits, talking to their babies, and being physically near them. As the baby's health improves, and tolerance for a bit more involvement is evident, parents are encouraged to take on more direct caregiving roles.

Involvement in the Level II Nursery

Babies in the level II nursery are more likely to be available to developmental care in general, especially when they "graduate" to room oxygen and are considered by the medical staff to be growers. The SLP may serve the infant's needs in the role of consultant to NICU staff and family members, providing information about oral stimulation; reducing tactile defensiveness in and around the baby's mouth; giving information on the benefits of nonnutritive sucking for babies who are tube fed; recognizing the baby's signs of stress and reducing interactional demands on the child during those periods; teaching the significance of eye contact between child and caregiver; and emphasizing the importance of talking to the child in a soothing, reassuring, pleasant manner. The SLP may also play the part of coach to the parent or designated caregiver, encouraging appropriate interactions or teaching about and demonstrating feeding techniques or strategies designed to build oral-motor coordination in preparation for oral feedings. The SLP may also participate in discharge planning by providing the family with lists of community contacts through which follow-up developmental monitoring and assessments are available and assisting in the design of a plan that assures a smooth transition from the structured world of the NICU to the home and community.

Obviously the SLP who works in the hospital setting needs a basic understanding of preterm infants and their problems. Likewise, it is the responsibility of the SLP to provide staff education that helps other members of the team understand the important relationship between an infant's very earliest experiences and subsequent communicative development.[9] Participation in staff-development seminars, on-site training provided by other members of the team, and participation in continuing-education programs to acquire and enhance skills are also required of the SLP.

The SLP's work is generally not to provide direct therapy to the infant but rather involves the processes of team functioning and the principles of adult education and interaction with members of the professional staff and parents.

The concept of interdisciplinary developmental care in the NICU is rapidly becoming the norm. VandenBerg[10] summarized the essential knowledge base required of NICU personnel: knowledge of normal infant development, knowledge of atypical infant development, and knowledge of family dynamics and functioning (pp. 163–164). Added specialized knowledge areas cited by VandenBerg include (1) knowledge of fetal and newborn brain development, (2) knowledge of medical conditions of premature and full-term neonates, (3) knowledge of neonatal preterm and full-term infant behaviors and development, (4) knowledge of ecology of the NICU, (5) knowledge of staffing patterns and the cultural patterns in the NICU, and (6) knowledge of parenting in the NICU. These areas of specialized knowledge clearly apply to personnel across all disciplines who function as members of the NICU team.

OTHER CONSIDERATIONS

There are some general considerations regarding work in the NICU with which the SLP must be familiar. These include information about infection control, characteristics of preterm infants, signs of infant stress, and roles of other members of the multidisciplinary team.

Infection Control

The NICU staff must observe strict infection-control protocols. Although the requirements vary somewhat from site to site, universal infection control precautions are common to all sites.

It is imperative that staff who contact the infants know and use appropriate hand-washing procedures. Before or upon entering the unit, hands are washed thoroughly, using a germicidal soap or solution and a scrub-brush or pad (paying special attention to the nails). Scrubs of 2–5 minutes are usually required. Rings should be removed (pinning them to scrub suit, apron, or undergarment with a safety pin to avoid potential loss or theft). Hands should be carefully washed between contacts with different infants and before a subsequent contact with a child if the staff member has handled equipment. Clean cloth gowns or disposable aprons customarily are worn by staff and visitors to the unit. Depending on hospital policy, latex gloves may also be required; they always should be used by workers who have a cut, burn, or other wound on the hand. Gloves should be changed between contacts with different babies and after handling equipment. Those SLPs who provide oral stimulation or participate in therapeutic feeding activities must be especially alert to the potential for spreading infection through improper hand washing and lax sanitary precautions.

The advent of congenital acquired immunodeficiency syndrome (AIDS) among newborn infants has made it imperative that certain additional precautions be taken by personnel. Some hospitals require masking and eye protection as a precaution against unanticipated exposure to urine, blood, or other body fluids. Although the SLP is less likely than the medical staff to have high-risk exposure, many AIDS babies have neurologic involvement that affects their developmental progress. Exposure to the virus is possible during assessment and intervention activities. The practitioner should be familiar with universal precautions for health care providers.[11]

Characteristics of Preterm Infants

Preterm infants (those born before 40 weeks' gestation by some definitions, or earlier than 38 weeks by the World Health Organization's definition) possess a number of common characteristics that have a bearing on development. An infant's gestational age can be established by a combination of means. The most commonly used measures include (1) date of birth from conception (9 months plus 1 week is a common reckoning of term); (2) birth weight (i.e., average, small, or large for gestational age); and (3) physical characteristics (i.e., presence or absence of lanugo [body hair], skin color and transparency or opaqueness, and reflexes). Preemies are often low birth weight (LBW; <1,500 g) or very low birth weight (VLBW; <1,000 g); and micropreemies can have birth weights of less than 800 g. The organ systems of preterm infants are immature, especially the respiratory system.

Preterm infants can require immediate—and sometimes heroic—treatment to sustain life. It is not uncommon for preterm infants with respiratory problems to receive surfactant therapy (prophylactically to prevent development of respiratory distress or therapeutically to treat established respiratory distress) and then to be on oxygen therapy for a period of time. Some infants experience bronchopulmonary dysplasia, a condition linked with developmental problems.[12] Depending on the circumstances, the oxygen requirements to sustain life can have deleterious effects on the child's hearing or vision, which, in turn, places the child at risk for subsequent difficulties in communicative development.

Many preterm infants suffer from hypoxia (inadequate supply of oxygen). They may also have episodes of apnea (cessation of breathing for 15 seconds or longer) for a short or prolonged period of time. Those who work with preterm infants and with infants who are admitted to the NICU for other reasons need to know that a bluish tinge to the lips, skin, or nails can be a sign that the child needs medical attention immediately.[4] However, these signs can be present in babies who are long-term oxygen dependent and are being treated for chronic hypoxia.

Other problems seen frequently in the NICU and implicated in developmental delays or disorders include (1) intraventricular hemorrhages (grades III and IV being significant), (2) prenatal drug exposure (cocaine and crack cocaine being especially important), (3) perinatal asphyxia (which may require "blow-by" oxygen supplementation at feedings, continuous oxygen saturation monitoring, provision of an apnea monitor at discharge, or any combination of these), (4) seizures, (5) fetal alcohol syndrome, (6) anatomic anomalies involving the head and neck, (7) congenital or perinatal infections, and (8) frank neuromotor impairment.

Signs of Infant Stress

Babies are adept at signaling their need to discontinue interactions with their caregivers. Unfortunately, not all caregivers are adept at reading the signals. The communicative disorders specialist should be alert to the infant's attempts to communicate a need to rest from the current activity, regardless of how passive the activity seems to the adult. The baby may exhibit one or a combination of the following signals that indicate stress:

- Yawning
- Averting eye contact
- Straightening the arms
- Stiffening the body
- Covering the face with a hand
- Gagging
- Spitting up
- Sneezing
- Spreading the fingers
- Arching the back
- Crying
- Saluting (arms up in the air)
- Coughing
- Changing color
- Abrupt changes in muscle tone
- Abrupt changes in respiratory rate
- Abrupt changes in heart rate
  Bradycardia (slowing)
  Tachycardia (racing)
- Apnea

The SLP needs to be aware of the superficial physical signs that are considered significant by the medical staff. McKenzie suggested a useful framework for

Table 5.1   Infant Cues to Behavioral Organization

Element	Organized	Disorganized
Color	Even Pink Stable	Uneven Pale, blue, or labile
Gaze	Focused Connected Intense	Glazed Dull Stunned
Alertness	Peaceful Content Bright	Irritable Fussy Grunting
Motor	Smooth Ballet-like Quiet	Jerky Erratic Staccato
Breathing	Regular	Irregular Colic

Source: Adapted from M McKenzie. How Do You Say CCMDFFSDS? Keynote address at Region IV Interagency Coordinating Council's Multidisciplinary Conference on Handicapped Infants and Toddlers, Lafayette, LA, October 1990.

identifying the level of behavioral organization in newborns, which is shown in Table 5.1.[13]

Sometimes the staff inadvertently creates stressful conditions for the fragile infant. For example, difficulty in maintaining appropriate body temperature is a common problem for preterm infants. Newborns do not shiver to maintain body temperature, and a great deal of energy is expended in re-establishing an adequate temperature after it has been lost. Preterm babies need their energy for other purposes. As simple as it may seem, the SLP (or other staff member) with cold hands should warm them before handling, positioning, or initiating stimulation activities with the infant.

Another inadvertent cause of infant stress can be related to excessive auditory stimulation of the preterm infant. Although a number of researchers have confirmed that appropriate auditory stimulation can have positive effects, cautions against overstimulation of any kind is a paramount consideration. Unless there is a current contraindication, it can be appropriate to suggest talking and singing to the baby, playing tape recordings of the mother's voice, and playing soft music. Babies who can tolerate these types of auditory stimuli have been shown to have higher scores on infant assessment tests and improved physical growth.[14–16]

The SLP must coordinate efforts with medical staff, other allied health professionals, and parents, who all interact with the infant at various times. Ongoing communication with the nursing staff assists the SLP in becoming acquainted with each infant's general condition, current status, temperament, feeding schedule, schedule of procedures or tests ordered for the day, and other important procedural information.

SPECIALIZED TEAMS IN THE NEONATAL INTENSIVE CARE UNIT

The preceding discussion provides an overview of the many people and specialty areas represented in the NICU in general. Each member of the team is important to optimizing care for children admitted to the NICU, and each member works in conjunction with the other members of the staff, contributing unique expertise and experience. In addition to the team in general, there are also smaller teams designed to meet specialized needs of the patients and their families and comprised of a smaller number of practitioners who usually also serve on the total NICU team.

Composition, Styles, and Roles for the Speech-Language Pathologist

In addition to the highly specialized team constituted by the NICU staff, specialized teams often bear titles that reflect the functions they perform. Examples of such teams include the following:

- Feeding teams can be composed of an occupational therapist, nurse, physician, nutritionist, SLP, and parent.
- Developmental assessment teams include specialists with expertise in sensorimotor, neurobehavioral, social, emotional, and communicative development. A growing number of multidisciplinary developmental assessment teams have been established as a result of implementation of early-intervention legislation. Under the Part C model (formerly Part H), parents are team members, along with professionals, serving as decision makers and contributing to the fund of knowledge about their child's individual development.
- Parent and family support teams sometimes exist for the purpose of providing information, support, and technical training to parents and other family members who are caregivers of infants discharged from the NICU. During the infant's hospital stay, parents may be introduced to families of unit "graduates," who assist them in anticipating what to expect when they take their baby home.
- Discharge planning teams provide the family with information and recommended procedures to implement the infant's care following release from the hospital. Discharge planning is often handled by a designated individual, generally a social worker or a nurse, but team planning is becoming more common. In some hospitals, all discharge planning for the NICU is handled through the multidisciplinary team.

- Follow-up teams conduct regular follow-up monitoring of NICU graduates. Though more often conducted in a clinic format, follow-up monitoring is sometimes provided in the home by an outreach team from the
  NICU. Studies indicate that developmental follow-up care is useful for
  preterm babies whose only problem is prematurity.[17]

Because communicative development is dependent on and interrelated
with development in other modalities, the SLP has much to offer as a member
of many specialized teams. The present focus on prevention and habilitation, as
opposed to the rehabilitative focus of the recent past, encourages a proactive
approach in identifying and using the infant's developing skills in one area to
build skills in related areas. Developmental intervention gives families objectives to work toward and emphasizes establishing positive outcomes, rather
than focusing on remedial activities designed to undo established behaviors.

Infant Assessment in the Neonatal Intensive Care Unit

Infants admitted to the NICU are assessed constantly. The purposes of the
assessments vary, but they usually analyze the child's physical state in relation to
survival and wellness. As noted earlier, babies in the NICU are exposed to a
great deal of stimulation. Their schedules are not the same as those followed by
infants who spend a brief period of time in the hospital and then go home to the
rhythms of family life. They must undergo treatments that in many cases are
aversive. They live in an environment in which the lights are always on and the
hustle and bustle of activity is constant. All of this must be taken into consideration as the SLP participates in assessments.

The SLP may provide or participate in providing at least two major assessments in the NICU: feeding assessments and developmental assessments, both of
which are performed as part of the team effort.

Feeding Assessment

Once the immediate medical problems have been resolved, concern shifts to the
child's ability to take in sufficient calories for growth and development. Many infants
initially receive nourishment intravenously. Oral feeding is the normal and preferred
means of feeding as soon as neuromotor development has advanced enough to make
it feasible. Some infants have great difficulty managing the motor coordination
required to feed from bottle or breast, and it is those children who require a feeding
assessment. There are any number of reasons a child can fail to develop a normal
suck-swallow pattern. Included on the list of possible reasons are the following:

- Prematurity
- Poor general health
- Lack of motor coordination
- Respiratory complications

- Cerebral palsy
- Unilateral vocal cord paralysis
- Paresis
- Hypotonia
- Neuromotor impairment
- Cardiac problems
- Cleft palate
- Other craniofacial anomalies

Because vegetative functions of the oral mechanism predate developmentally and form the foundation for later functions of oral communication, it is entirely appropriate for a knowledgeable SLP to be a part of the feeding assessment team. Good nutrition promotes growth and development in all areas, including cognitive, social, and communicative development. Overt and submucous palatal clefts and other craniofacial anomalies that are associated with poor oral feeding can also lead to communicative impairment. Suggestions for conducting feeding assessments for infants and toddlers along with selected techniques to assist in development of appropriate oral motor and feeding skills are included in Appendix A. It must be reiterated that the SLP who participates in or conducts feeding and swallowing assessment must have adequate training to do so.

Developmental Assessment

A discussion of the general nature of multidisciplinary developmental assessment is provided above. The present discussion is designed to provide additional information pertinent to working with medical and allied health specialists on their turf, that is, the hospital. Remembering that their primary orientation and training have focused on sustaining life and curing disease, the developmental assessment will probably be approached by the medical staff from an orientation toward physical growth and neurologic development. There may be an established protocol for conducting such assessments, using developmental assessment tools that are familiar to the medical staff. Increasingly, developmental assessments are being performed by physical therapists, occupational therapists, or both and nursing staff trained to conduct them. Suggested changes in their usual methods of completing evaluations may not be received well and should be approached with caution. It may be more appropriate to suggest including an additional element in the assessment to address early communication development. Modifications in the interdisciplinary assessment procedure can emerge as mutual recommendations after the SLP becomes a trusted member of the team.

Developmental tests with which the medical community is most likely to be familiar are shown in Table 5.2. It is essential to know how the norms were developed for the tests in use in a particular unit. For example, for the Bayley Scales, typically developing children between 2 and 30 months living at home were the "norming" population. Healthy newborns were also used in developing the Neonatal Behavioral Assessment Scale. Instruments normed on infants not known

Table 5.2 Assessment Instruments Commonly Used in Infant Assessments

Tool	Reference	Comments
The Neonatal Behavioral Assessment Scale (NBAS)	22	This is a widely used tool recommended for full-term newborns or preterm infants 37-weeks postconception and in stable medical condition. Administration time is approximately 30 minutes.
The Assessment of Preterm Infant Behavior	23	This tool was designed to be a downward extension of the NBAS. Examiners must be carefully trained in its administration. Assessment time is approximately 30 minutes.
Naturalistic Observation of the Preterm Neonate	24	This is an observation method that focuses on preterm newborns' responses to stress and adjustments in response to environmental supports. System requires observing the infant in 2-minute time segments, and reports require anecdotal notes of the examiner.

to have disabilities and who were born at term have obvious limitations in their application to other populations.

Many hospitals' and some individual states' early-intervention systems (e.g., Louisiana, see Appendix A, Figure A.2) have adopted protocols based on the philosophical and procedural protocols of several instruments that their practitioners find particularly useful.

Observation of the child's patterns of development over a period of time; review of chart entries, medical information, and specific neurodevelopmental assessments; and discussions with staff and parents make it possible to gather assessment information without being intrusive or disturbing the baby. If the baby appears to be having problems with markers of communicative development, discussions with the staff can include seeking technical information from them with regard to the possible causes of the problem and management options, as well as providing information for their consideration from the perspective of speech-language pathology.

Working with Families in the Neonatal Intensive Care Unit

The necessity of dealing with families and their feelings in an empathetic and constructive way is stressed throughout this book. Very few families anticipate having an infant with problems. Parents struggle with their feelings of grief over the loss of the perfect child whom they were prepared to receive, feelings of concern and anxiety about the survival or appearance of the child who was born, feelings of helplessness and concern about lacking basic information on their child's condition, feelings of apprehension about the decisions they are required to make (often under extreme pressure to make them quickly), and the anxieties and stress brought about by the financial aspects of their situation.[18,19] In such a situation, it is counterproductive to flood the family with information that they are not ready to accept. The best-intentioned SLP who approaches the family too soon and overwhelms them with information or suggestions about behavioral or attitudinal changes is doomed to failure. Moreover, the family may erect emotional barriers that have an adverse effect on future interactions and make it difficult to develop an effective intervention plan.

The family's desire for additional information, their ability to process new knowledge, and their interest in pursuing developmental enhancements becomes clear to the SLP who employs active listening techniques and is appropriately responsive to the family's needs as *they* express them. The family's priorities change, sometimes several times in a single day, as they process the information they are receiving from a myriad of sources. There are always primary and secondary issues about which they are concerned. Individual members of the family vary in their levels of acceptance, capacity to cope with the various stresses connected with their infant's care and nurturing, and in their desire for specific guidance from professionals. Appreciating the dynamics of each family's situation and dealing with each situation individually is a team effort.

For these reasons, questions such as "How may I help you today?" or "Is there anything I can do to help with that?" are always preferable to statements such as "Let me tell you what I think you should focus on next" or "Let me show you how to get your baby to do [or stop doing] that." Rossetti suggested asking "What has changed since we last talked?" as a way of obtaining information, conveying genuine interest, and orienting the interaction toward issues about which the parents, rather than the SLP, are concerned.[1]

Assisting parents in knowing what to expect is another way to help them focus their questions about their interactions with the infant. For example, the SLP can tell the parents that consistent interactive responses from their baby are unlikely to appear before 28 weeks' gestational age. That knowledge, combined with an understanding that an otherwise healthy, premature baby who is held and talked to generally gains weight faster[1,20] and can recognize the mother's voice can cause parents to increase their visits and time spent holding the baby. The infant's early passivity is less worrisome when parents know that it is expected.[20]

As Rocco[21] observed,

[a]ssessments shape expectations. That is why they are so powerful. Assessments of infants and toddlers have a profound effect on how parents view their children's future and how they view their own competence as parents. Professionals who are involved in the assessment of very young

children's development need to be aware of the power of the process and must be careful not to abuse it (p. 55).

Payment for Services Rendered

Billings for services rendered can be indirect (i.e., billed to an insurer or state agency) or direct (i.e., charged to the parent responsible for paying the baby's hospital bill). Billing can be done automatically as part of the NICU package provided by the hospital or can be accomplished through itemized charges submitted by the professional who renders service.

It is important that the SLP find out what is reimbursable under the various mechanisms and the appropriate codes or terminology used to access the reimbursement source. For example, neurodevelopmental assessments, usually conducted by the physical or occupational therapist, are commonly reimbursable. Communication assessments, less familiar to insurers of children in this age group, may or may not be considered reimbursable as a unitary billing item. They have, however, traditionally been an appropriate portion of the pediatric developmental assessment (see the communication oral language assessment sections of standardized developmental assessment tools) and, as such, are regularly reimbursed. Wording is often critical to whether a claim is reimbursed or denied—a fact of life in any area of health care, but one with which the SLP who is inexperienced in reimbursement practices may lack familiarity

Many early-intervention services are now covered under Medicaid, which has also recently revised its eligibility requirements to include families with higher income levels than were eligible before. Familiarity with Medicaid reimbursement policies is important for practitioners who work in any hospital or other setting that serves Medicaid-eligible families.

SUMMARY

Specialized skills and evolving roles for the SLP in the NICU constitute a relatively new and challenging aspect of professional practice. Those SLPs who deal with infants after their hospital discharge must also have an appreciation for the NICU experience that was so recently an important part of the life of both baby and family.

REFERENCES

1. Rossetti LM. Speech-Language Pathologists in the NICU. Paper presented at ASHA Conference, St. Louis, November 1989.
2. Brazelton TB. A Window on the Newborn's World: More Than Two Decades of Experience with the Neonatal Behavioral Assessment Scale. In SJ Meisels, E Fenichel (eds), New Visions for the Developmental Assessment of Infants and Young Children. Washington, DC: Zero to Three, 1996;127.
3. Gottwald WR, Alper BS. Neonatal Intensive Care: The Speech-Language Pathologist's Role. Paper presented at ASHA Conference, St. Louis, November 1989.

4. Harrison H, Kositsky A. The Premature Baby Book: A Parents' Guide to Coping and Caring in the First Years. New York: St. Martin's Press, 1983.
5. Clark DL, Copradero L, Goss KC, Manos D. Effects of rocking on neuromuscular development in the premature. Biol Neonate 1989;56:306.
6. Gorski PA. Premature Infant Behavioral and Physiological Responses to Caregiving Interventions in an Intensive Care Nursery. In J Call, E Galenson, R Tyson (eds), Frontiers of Infant Psychiatry. New York: Basic Books, 1982;256.
7. Mouradian LE, Als H. The influence of neonatal intensive care unit caregiving practices on motor functioning of preterm infants. Special issue: neonatal intensive care unit. Am J Occup Ther 1994;48:527.
8. Rauh VA, Nurcombe B, Achenbach T, Howell CT. The mother-infant transaction program. The content and implications of an intervention for the mothers of low-birthweight infants. Clin Perinatol 1990;17:31.
9. Miller RM, Groher ME. Medical Speech Pathology. Rockville, MD: Aspen, 1990.
10. VandenBerg MA. Basic competencies to begin developmental care in the intensive care nursery. Infants Young Child 1993;6:52.
11. American Speech-Language-Hearing Association, Committee on Quality Assurance. AIDS/HIV: implications for speech-language pathologists and audiologists. ASHA 1989;31:33.
12. Landry SH, Chapieski ML, Richardson MA, et al. The social competence of children born prematurely: effects of medical compilations and parent behaviors. Child Dev 1990;61:1605.
13. McKenzie M. How Do You Say CCMDFFSDS? Keynote address at Region IV Interagency Coordinating Council's Multidisciplinary Conference on Handicapped Infants and Toddlers, Lafayette, LA, October 1990.
14. Leib SA, Benefield DG, Greidubaldi J. Effects of early intervention and stimulation of the preterm infant. Pediatrics 1980;66:83.
15. Katz V. Auditory stimulation and developmental behavior of the premature infant. Nurs Res 1971;20:196.
16. Kramer LI, Pierpoint ME. Rocking waterbeds and auditory stimuli to enhance the growth of preterm infants. J Pediatr 1976;88:297.
17. Ramey CT, Bryant DM, Wasik BH, et al. Infant health and development program for low birth weight premature infants: program elements, family participation, and child intelligence. Pediatrics 1992;89:454.
18. Minde K, Trehub S, Corter G, et al. Mother-child relationships in the premature nursery: an observational study. Pediatrics 1978;61:373.
19. Popper BK. Achieving Change in Assessment Practices: A Parent's Perspective. In SJ Meisels, E Fenichel (eds), New Visions for the Developmental Assessment of Infants and Young Children. Washington, DC: Zero to Three, 1996;59.
20. Moore ML. High-Risk Mothers and Infants. Presented at the seminar sponsored by the Woman's Foundation, Inc. Lafayette, LA, March 1988.
21. Rocco S. Toward Shared Commitment and Shared Responsibility: A Parent's Vision of Developmental Assessment. In SJ Meisels, E Fenichel (eds), New Visions for the Developmental Assessment of Infants and Young Children. Washington, DC: Zero to Three, 1996;55.
22. Brazelton TB. Neonatal Behavioral Assessment Scale. Clinics in Developmental Medicine, no. 88. London: Spastics International Medical Publisher, 1984.
23. Als H, Lester BM, Tronick E, Brazelton TB. Manual for the Assessment of Preterm Infant Behavior (APIB). In HE Fitzgerald, BM Lester, MW Yogman (eds), Theory and Research in Behavioral Pediatrics (Vol. 1). New York: Plenum, 1983.
24. Als H. A Manual for the Naturalistic Observation of the Newborn (Preterm and Fullterm) [rev]. Boston: Harvard Medical School, Department of Psychiatry, 1984.

6

Identification and Assessment of Hearing-Impaired Infants and Toddlers

Thomas G. Rigo and Shalini Arehole

Hearing evaluation of infants and toddlers is one of the most challenging aspects of the practice of audiology. Many of the test procedures are unique to this population and must be tailored to the child's particular capabilities. The audiologist's primary goal is the identification and comprehensive assessment of the infant's hearing impairment at as young an age as possible. This is because it is necessary to obtain an accurate and detailed description of the degree and nature of the hearing loss before optimal hearing aid fitting and aural habilitation procedures can be initiated. As in adult assessment, the examiner must rely on a battery of test results to form a meaningful picture of the child's auditory capabilities. This battery includes both behavioral and objective tests that, when used in combination, provide information concerning the extent, site, and perceptual effect of the auditory pathology. This chapter reviews the procedures that are commonly used in test centers today and will provide the reader some insight into the capabilities and limitations of the techniques described.

BEHAVIORAL THRESHOLD ASSESSMENT

Neonates

Behavioral assessment of neonates is limited to observations of overt reflexive responses to sound. Optimally, the infant is tested in a state of light sleep to minimize the false-positives that occur with awake babies and the false-negatives likely with infants in deep sleep.[1] However, in light of the reality of the test situation and the transitory nature of states of arousal, evaluation should be attempted regardless of the initial state observed.

The neonate is most responsive to complex, wide-band, sudden-onset stimuli.[2] White noise, narrow-band noise, speech bursts (e.g., *buh-buh-buh*), and premeasured noisemakers (e.g., squeeze toys or horns) are good examples. Suprathreshold stimulation is necessary to elicit observable and reliable responses. During the first several weeks of life, responses to sound include

101

arousal from sleep, eye widening, eye blinks, startling, changes in respiratory pattern, and initiation or cessation of the sucking reflex.[3] The type of response demonstrated by the infant is dependent on the prestimulus state. Quiet and sleeping babies show increases in activity; active babies display reductions or cessation of prestimulus behaviors.[4]

The probability and validity of response are highest when testing is conducted in a sound-treated audiometric booth. Examinations can be administered in a quiet room, provided ambient noise levels do not exceed 60 dB SPL.[1] Testing is usually conducted with the child in the parent's arms. The tester and parent should ensure that the child's ears remain unobstructed. The stimulus should be presented briefly (for 2 seconds), and the response must be seen within 2 seconds of stimulus presentation. If noisemakers are used, they should be held motionless next to the child for several seconds before stimulation, and any airstream emitted from the noisemaker should be directed away from the child. Repeat testing should be conducted to validate the initial response. Most examiners conclude testing by introducing an intense stimulus; the clear startle response that is usually seen serves to substantiate the more subtle responses observed with softer stimuli. Testing with frequency-specific stimuli (e.g., warble tones, narrow-band noise) can be attempted, but the examiner should be aware of the infant's relatively low responsiveness to these stimuli and the probability of the response ceasing to manifest on repeated stimulation. Information relative to type of hearing loss can be obtained by repeating the above procedures with a bone-conduction receiver placed high on the infant's forehead and comparing these responses to those observed in response to air-conducted stimuli.

Older Infants

By 3 months of age, the infant's developing auditory experience and motoric maturation allow for more elaborate orienting responses to sound. At 3–4 months, orientation is limited to a horizontal head turn towards the sound source. Initially, infants localize horizontally to sounds originating at, above, and below their eye level. As motor control improves, more accurate localizations emerge. Direct localizations to sounds below eye level are seen by 9–13 months and above eye level by 13–16 months.[1]

The signal intensity necessary to elicit a behavioral response decreases in a systematic fashion as the infant grows. Table 6.1 presents an index detailing the stimulus levels needed to produce a response in normal-hearing infants. Two trends are of particular importance. First, the growing infant responds to decreasing sound intensities irrespective of the type of stimulus presented. Second, at any age, the infant remains most responsive to complex, relevant stimuli, such as speech.

The child's increased responsiveness to sound provides the examiner with the opportunity to acquire more detailed sensitivity data. Of prime importance is the determination of behavioral thresholds for frequency-specific stimuli. Use of wide-band inputs provides little information about hearing sensitivity as a

Table 6.1 Auditory Behavior Index for Infants

Age	Noisemakers (Approximate SPL)	Warble Tones (HL)	Speech (HL)	Startle to Speech
0–6 wks	50–70 dB	75 dB	40–60 dB	65 dB
6 wks–4 mos	50–60 dB	70 dB	45 dB	65 dB
4–7 mos	40–50 dB	50 dB	20 dB	65 dB
7–9 mos	30–40 dB	45 dB	15 dB	65 dB
9–13 mos	25–35 dB	38 dB	10 dB	65 dB
13–16 mos	25–30 dB	30 dB	5 dB	65 dB
16–24 mos	25 dB	25 dB	5 dB	65 dB

Source: Reprinted with permission from JL Northern, MP Downs. Hearing in Children (4th ed). Baltimore: Williams & Wilkins, 1991;145.

function of frequency. An infant's audiometric configuration can be established only with frequency-specific inputs such as warble tones or, to a lesser extent, narrow-band noise. For example, an infant who suffers from high-frequency hearing loss responds to a simple speech stimulus, such as *buh-buh-buh*, at normal threshold by receiving and reacting to the low-frequency energy contained within the syllable *buh*. The response indicates that at least some portion of the child's hearing is within normal range but does not rule out the presence of hearing loss.

The use of frequency-specific stimuli in infant testing presents a problem of response habituation. A significant number of stimuli must be introduced during a test session to acquire sensitivity data across a meaningful range of frequencies. Unfortunately, inputs such as warble tones are abstract and nonmeaningful, and an infant's response to these types of sounds extinguishes quickly. This difficulty can be overcome by using a test technique most frequently referred to as *visual reinforcement audiometry* (VRA).[5] In this operant conditioning procedure, a visual stimulus serves to reinforce the infant's localization response to sound. Reinforcers can range from blinking lights to animated toy animals. In effect, the entertaining visual event following a response to an auditory signal sustains the continued reaction to that signal.

The VRA procedure is best conducted with the infant facing forward on the parent's lap. Stimuli are presented from one of two speakers located 45–90 degrees to each side of the child's position and introduced at descending intensity levels until a threshold is reached. Some infants, particularly those younger than 12 months, respond inconsistently to warble tones despite the best attempts of the examiner. In these cases, introduction of narrow-band noises, music, noisemakers, or speech can provide better results. It must be remembered, however, that these types of inputs limit, to varying degrees, one's ability to determine audiometric configuration because of the loss of frequency specificity.

Soundfield testing is generally considered the most appropriate method of evaluating children under 2 years of age. The great majority of children in this age group do not tolerate placement of earphones, and their attempted use often results in aggravated test situations. Soundfield procedures, however, impose several limitations on test interpretation. First, depending on age, infants with severe and profound hearing loss may not show any response in a soundfield test environment, thus limiting the examiner's ability to differentiate these degrees of impairment. This is because of the output limitations of soundfield systems, which, for example, can range from 90 to 105 dB HL for speech inputs. Second, conclusions concerning individual ear sensitivity can be reached only when testing is conducted with earphones. It is incorrect to assume that the observation of accurate localizations during soundfield testing implies bilateral sensitivity. It follows that the examiner can only assume that the better ear is being tested when assessment is limited to soundfield procedures. Finally, the inability to determine bone-conduction thresholds in soundfield prevents the examiner from ascertaining whether a measured hearing loss is conductive, sensorineural, or mixed in nature.

Modification of the standard soundfield procedure can be attempted with headphones and the bone vibrator. The success of these procedures is, of course, dependent on the child's willingness to allow placement of these devices. Localizations can be successfully generalized from soundfield to headphone conditions.[6] When testing with the bone vibrator, however, the examiner should accept any visual response observed because localizations can be difficult or impossible to achieve or, in some cases, can be reversed due to the occlusion effect.

2- to 3-Year-Old Children

By 2 years of age, children may begin to respond successfully to more conventional threshold procedures. The technique of choice for the 2- to 3-year-old child is conditioned-play audiometry. In this procedure, the child is conditioned to respond to an auditory signal with some form of play activity, such as putting pegs in a hole, throwing blocks into a bucket, stacking rings on a stick, or putting pieces of a puzzle together. Conditioned play should be attempted on all children older than 2 years of age, but the procedure may not be entirely successful for many children between the ages of 2 and 3 years. Levels of success are highly dependent on the child's disposition, manageability, social maturity, and cognitive and language abilities. By 3 years of age, however, the procedure is usually effective for all children but those most difficult to test.

Play audiometry begins with a conditioning period in which the child is trained to perform the play activity in response to the suprathreshold presentation of a pure tone. Most children respond appropriately to verbal instruction and encouragement; for younger children and those with cognitive or receptive language limitations, however, it is usually necessary for the examiner to shape the response. After conditioning, testing is conducted with earphones and the bone vibrator using conventional threshold-seeking techniques.

SPEECH AUDIOMETRY

Speech audiometrics should be considered a routine component of the pediatric hearing evaluation. For children younger than 3 years of age, procedures are restricted in scope and usually are conducted in an informal and subjective manner because of the infant's limited responsiveness, short attention span, and restricted receptive vocabulary. Despite these constraints, speech testing is often the only procedure that can be administered successfully to a young child who is difficult to test. Speech materials are more meaningful and interesting than inputs such as warble tones and bands of noise and usually hold a child's attention for a longer period of time.

Speech Detection Threshold

Speech detection threshold refers to the lowest intensity at which a listener can detect the presence of a speech stimulus. It is an awareness measure and does not necessarily imply recognition or comprehension of the stimulus. It is usually the sole speech measure obtainable for infants younger than 1 year due to their limited linguistic development.

Speech Reception Threshold

Speech reception threshold (SRT) is generally thought of as the softest intensity at which speech can be recognized. It is defined operationally as the lowest intensity level at which a listener can repeat 50% of speech stimuli presented. The SRT is usually determined by presenting spondee words in isolation. It has been found to be highly correlated to midfrequency pure-tone average in cases of flat and mildly sloping hearing loss.[7] SRT can be acquired in older infants after some degree of receptive language has been established.

Word Recognition

Word recognition (also referred to as *speech discrimination*) is the ability to identify monosyllabic words when presented in isolation. The specific test procedure depends on the type of information that is being sought. Testing is usually conducted to determine the listener's maximum intelligibility score. In this procedure, a list of 25 or 50 stimulus items is presented at a sensation level of 40 dB (re: SRT), and a percent-correct recognition score is obtained. The test results can be helpful in determining lesion site, predicting the benefits to be obtained from using a hearing aid, and identifying the specific linguistic confusions caused by the impairment.

Standardized word-recognition tests for children younger than 2.5 years of age are not generally available. The assessment of word intelligibility for these children is informal, with the stimulus items and response tasks shaped to meet the child's level of function. Standardized tests include the Northwestern

University–Children's Perception of Speech test[8] for children older than 2.5 years of age, the Auditory Numbers Test[9] and the Pediatric Speech Intelligibility test[10] for children at least 3 years of age, and the Word Intelligibility by Picture Identification test[11] for children between 4 and 6 years of age. These ages refer to receptive language age. Most standardized tests use closed-stimulus sets and picture-identification response modes.

IMMITTANCE TESTING

The immittance battery consists of two tests: tympanometry and acoustic reflex testing. These tests are designed to evaluate the status and function of the middle ear and the acoustic reflex arc, respectively. The main feature of the immittance meter is the probe assembly and its three measurement systems. The first system, consisting of a sound generator and loudspeaker, emits a low-frequency pure tone (referred to as the probe tone) of fixed intensity and frequency. High-frequency probe tones can also be used to gain additional information about certain types of middle-ear pathologies. The second system is composed of an air pump and manometer, which serve to alter and measure the air pressure within the ear canal. Most immittance meters provide for pressure variations within the range of +300 to –600 daPa. The third system consists of a microphone that measures the SPL within the external meatus. Before testing, a pliable probe tip is placed over the end of the probe assembly and inserted into the ear canal so that an airtight seal is obtained.

The central measure in immittance testing is middle-ear admittance. In practice, admittance refers to the mobility, or vibratory efficiency, of the middle-ear structures. It is derived from the measurement of the SPL contained within the sealed meatal cavity and is expressed in cubic centimeter (cc) or milliliter (ml) units of equivalent volume. The relationship among these three measures is complex and is best explained within the context of the tympanometric test technique.

Tympanometry

Normal transmission of sound through the conductive system is dependent on the vibration of the tympanic membrane and ossicles of the middle ear. The admittance of the middle-ear system is greatest when air pressure is equal on each side of the tympanic membrane. Any pressure imbalance between the outer and middle ear displaces the tympanic membrane from its normal position. This displacement reduces the membrane's ability to vibrate in response to sound energy, resulting in a reduction in the admittance of the conductive system. Other factors that can affect middle-ear admittance include the presence of fluid or other material in the middle-ear space, a stiffening or a disarticulation of the ossicular chain, and structural damage to or changes in the elasticity of the tympanic membrane.

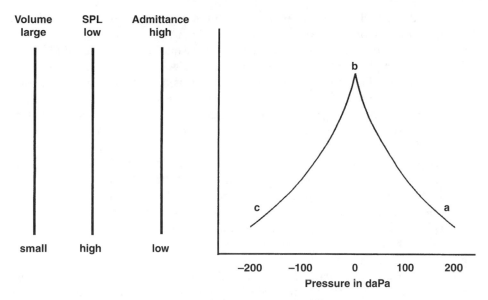

Figure 6.1   The relationship among the measures of middle-ear admittance, sound pressure level (SPL) in the external meatus, and equivalent volume in a normal middle ear.

In tympanometry, the admittance of the middle ear is measured as air pressure is varied in the external meatus. A normal tympanogram and the way in which it is derived are shown in Figure 6.1. Tympanometry begins by inducing a positive pressure of 200 daPa in the external meatus (Figure 6.1, point *a*), creating a pressure imbalance across the tympanic membrane. The imbalance displaces and stiffens the membrane, reducing middle-ear admittance. As a result, a large proportion of the acoustic energy of the probe tone is reflected from the tympanic membrane and back into the ear canal. Under this condition, the probe microphone measures a high SPL within the external meatus. The air pressure is then reduced, lessening the imbalance across the tympanic membrane. When the air pressure in the external meatus is equal to that in the middle ear (Figure 6.1, point *b*), the admittance of the middle ear system is maximized. A large proportion of the acoustic energy of the probe tone is transduced and passed through the middle ear, minimizing the level of reflected sound in the ear canal. At this point, the microphone measures a low SPL within the external meatus. As the pressure is reduced further (Figure 6.1, point *c*), a pressure imbalance is created again across the tympanic membrane. The membrane stiffens and admittance is reduced. The amount of reflected energy increases and, again, a high SPL is measured in the ear canal. As can be seen, the examiner can make inferences about the admittance of the middle ear by measuring the SPL within the external canal. The relationship is an inverse one; a high SPL is measured when middle-ear admittance is low, and a low SPL is measured when the admittance of the middle ear is high.

Middle-ear admittance is expressed in ml or cc units of equivalent volume. Under conditions of reduced admittance, the high SPL measured by the probe microphone is equivalent to that expected for a small cavity. When middle-ear admittance is high, the low SPL measured is equivalent to that expected for a larger cavity (see Figure 6.1). It is important to remember that changes in equivalent volume during tympanometry represent changes in the admittance of the middle-ear system, not in the physical volume of the external meatus. Equivalent volume measures correspond to actual cavity size only when the middle ear is noncompliant.

Two primary measures are used to classify and interpret tympanometric configurations: middle-ear pressure and static admittance. Middle-ear pressure is derived from the location of the admittance peak. Because admittance is maximal when pressure is equal in the outer and middle ear, pressure in the middle ear can be deduced as equal to that contained in the outer ear when peak admittance is reached. Middle-ear pressure is considered to be normal when it is ±100 daPa (0 daPa represents ambient pressure). Static admittance is computed by subtracting the volume reading at +200 daPa (point of lowest admittance) from the volume reading at the admittance peak (point of highest admittance). This is simply a way to quantify the mobility of the middle-ear system. A small static admittance value suggests a stiff middle ear, whereas a high value indicates a hypermobile, or flaccid, system. Normal static admittance values generally range between 0.3 ml and 1.6 ml for most instruments.

The most common tympanometric classification system is that described by Jerger.[12] The various configurations are shown in Figure 6.2. Included in the figure is an unclassified tympanogram that is usually referred to as *transitional* or *intermediate*. It is characterized by a shallow, rounded admittance peak occurring within or outside of the normal pressure range. Table 6.2 outlines the interpretive measures and associated conditions for each tympanometric configuration.

Tympanometry is of limited diagnostic value for infants younger than 7 months of age, because of high false-negative findings.[13] For these children, a flat configuration is strongly associated with a pathologic condition, but a normal result does not necessarily imply the absence of middle-ear involvement. Despite this limitation, tympanometry should be administered to this population in light of the incidence and consequence of middle-ear pathology during the first year of life.

Acoustic Reflex Testing

The *acoustic reflex* refers to the contraction of the stapedius muscle of the middle ear in response to an intense auditory stimulus. The action of the stapedius muscle is controlled by the facial nerve (cranial nerve VII) and a central network, or arc, located in the lower brain stem. The ipsilateral and contralateral pathways of the reflex arc give the acoustic reflex a bilateral character. That is, auditory stimulation to one ear elicits a stapedial contraction in both ears.

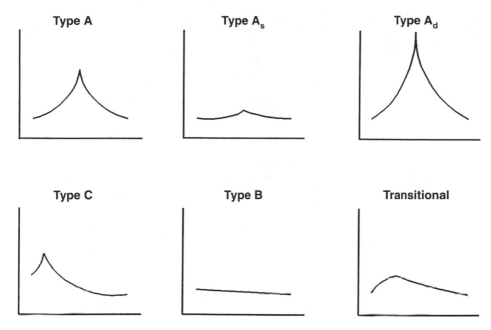

Figure 6.2   Classification of tympanometric configurations.

Contraction of the stapedius muscle causes a stiffening of the ossicular chain and a reduction in the admittance of the middle-ear system. Consequently, the acoustic reflex can be identified indirectly by the probe system as a change in the admittance of the middle ear on auditory stimulation. Because the reflex occurs bilaterally, it can be measured in the ear being stimulated (ipsilateral measurement) or in the ear contralateral to stimulation (contralateral measurement).

In acoustic-reflex assessment, the examiner measures the reflex threshold at octave frequencies of 500–4,000 Hz. The acoustic-reflex threshold is found normally at sensation levels of 70–100 dB. It is important to note that reflex thresholds are documented in HL values but are interpreted according to the sensation levels (re: audiometric threshold) at which they occur. Pathology is indicated when reflexes are absent or when their thresholds are found at sensation levels lower or higher than the normal range of 70–100 dB. By analyzing findings across test conditions, lesion sites can be localized to the conductive system, cochlea, auditory nerve, or facial nerve.

Reflex results are broadly classified into two groups: probe effects and stimulus effects. A *probe effect* refers to the presence of abnormal findings when the probe is placed in a particular ear, regardless of the ear being stimulated. A probe effect indicates either the presence of middle-ear pathology in the probe ear or the presence of a facial-nerve lesion medial to stapedial innervation.

A *stimulus effect* is indicated when reflex abnormalities are associated with stimulation to a particular ear, regardless of the ear in which the reflex is mea-

Table 6.2 Tympanometric Classifications and Associated Pathologic Conditions

Classification	Interpretive Measures	Associated Conditions
Type A	Normal pressure Normal admittance	Normal middle ear Otosclerosis
Type A$_s$	Normal pressure Reduced admittance	Otosclerosis Adhesions Tympanosclerosis Cholesteatoma
Type A$_d$	Normal pressure Elevated admittance	Disarticulation Flaccid tympanic membrane
Type C	Negative pressure Normal admittance	Eustachian tube dysfunction

Type B	No discernible peak
	Reduced admittance
		Effusion
		Cholesteatoma
		Foreign bodies
		Impacted cerumen
		Tympanic membrane
		  perforation (with
		  high volume)
		PE tubes in situ

Transitional	Shallow, rounded peak Normal or reduced admittance	Effusion Cholesteatoma

sured. Stimulus effects suggest pathology of the ascending (auditory) portion of the reflex arc and can be reliably determined only when measurement is made from a normal middle ear. The site of lesion within the auditory system can be established by analyzing the sensation levels at which the reflex thresholds occur.

Reflex thresholds at reduced sensation levels (<70 dB) indicate cochlear site of pathology. Reflex thresholds at elevated sensation levels (>100 dB) suggest neural pathology. In conductive losses, reflex thresholds occur at normal sensation levels, but the hearing levels may be higher than expected for a normal ear, as a result of the elevation of audiometric thresholds. Reflexes are absent under all test conditions in cases of bilateral conductive pathology, because the bilateral involvement prevents the measurement of reflexes in either ear.

OTOACOUSTIC EMISSIONS

Otoacoustic emissions (OAEs) are sounds generated by a normal cochlea during auditory processing. The emissions are soft and occur at subthreshold levels. It is believed that OAEs are produced by the electromotility of the outer hair cells. The OAEs generated within the cochlea travel through the middle ear and into the ear canal, where they can be measured with an insert microphone.

Any pathology that affects normal outer hair-cell activity reduces or abolishes the OAE response. This allows OAEs to be used to assess cochlear function.

There are two basic categories of OAEs being measured for clinical purposes: transient evoked otoacoustic emissions (TEOAEs) and distortion-product otoacoustic emissions (DPOAEs). TEOAEs are generated by introducing a short-duration stimulus to the ear.[14] DPOAEs are generated by a simultaneous presentation of two different tonal stimuli to the ear. Both OAE measures are well-suited to the infant population because they are reliable, rapid, cost-effective, and noninvasive.[14,15]

Transient-Evoked Otoacoustic Emissions

TEOAEs are recorded by presenting repeated click stimuli to the ear in a quiet environment. A click is a short, broadband stimulus with an instantaneous rise and fall time. The clicks are introduced through an eartip at a high intensity level (around 80 dB SPL). A microphone enclosed in the eartip records both ambient noise and the emissions generated by the cochlea. The amplitude of the emissions are extremely small compared to that of the noise. The repeated presentation of the click stimulus, however, increases the amplitude of the emissions and decreases the amplitude of the noise, allowing the visualization of the TEOAE. Typically, the TEOAE is seen over and above the background noise across the frequency range of 500–5,000 Hz.

TEOAEs are larger in infants than in adults.[16] Generally, infants' emissions are seen across a wider range of frequencies and at higher amplitudes. The differences in the response between infants and adults have been attributed to the difference in the dimensions of the ear canal, the angle of the tympanic membrane with respect to the ear canal, and the tissue composition of the ear canal.[17]

It is well established that TEOAEs are present in nonpathologic ears with hearing thresholds better than 20–30 dB HL.[15,18] In contrast, emissions are absent in listeners with hearing loss ranging from mild to profound.

In evaluating the TEOAE, the examiner takes into consideration the following factors: (1) the amplitude of the TEOAE versus that of ambient noise (signal-to-noise ratio), (2) the frequencies at which the emissions are present, and (3) the reproducibility of the response. Figure 6.3A shows the TEOAE test results of a normal-hearing patient. The emissions are clearly visible above the noise floor across frequencies 500–5,000 Hz. Figure 6.3B shows the TEOAE results of a patient with a sensorineural hearing loss at frequencies above 2,000 Hz. The absence of emissions above 2,000 Hz is indicative of hearing thresholds greater than 20–30 dB HL at these frequencies. However, the degree of hearing loss at these frequencies cannot be determined from TEOAE testing.

Distortion-Product Otoacoustic Emissions

DPOAEs are produced by the simultaneous presentation of two pure tones (called primary tones) that differ in frequency.[19] When the primary tones are

Figure 6.3 Transient evoked otoacoustic emissions (TEOAE) of a normal-hearing patient (A) and a patient with sensorineural hearing loss above 2,000 Hz (B). TEOAE response is shown in black; noise floor is shown in gray. (SNR = signal-to-noise ratio.)

introduced to the ear at a moderate intensity (60–70 dB SPL), they produce an emission with a frequency different from that of the two primary tones. This emission is referred to as the *distortion product*. The presence of the distortion product indicates normal cochlear function at the geometrical mean frequency of the primary tones. By shifting the frequencies of the primary tones and measuring the resultant distortion products, a measure of cochlear function across a range of frequencies can be obtained. A response is said to be present if DPOAE amplitudes are greater than the noise floor by at least 3 dB.[20] DPOAEs are present at frequencies whose hearing thresholds are within normal range. Emission amplitudes are reduced when hearing thresholds are between 15 and 50 dB HL. DPOAEs are not detected when hearing thresholds are greater than 50 dB HL. Figure 6.4A shows the DPOAE test results of the same patient as shown in Figure 6.3A. The emissions are seen to occur at least 3 dB above the noise floor across frequencies 1,000–6,000 Hz. Figure 6.4B shows the DPOAE results of the same patient as shown in Figure 6.3B. The absence of emissions above 2,000 Hz indicates sensorineural hearing loss at these frequencies.

Although evoked otoacoustic emissions (EOAE) show great promise as an objective and reliable test of cochlear function, there are several limitations to the procedure: (1) External or middle ear involvement can interfere with measurement of emissions and, therefore, abnormal results under these conditions do not necessarily indicate cochlear pathology; (2) a high level of ambient noise, such as that found in nurseries or neonatal intensive care units, can interfere with the measurement of emissions, particularly in the lower frequencies; and (3) neural involvement can adversely effect cochlear function and, consequently, the use of OAEs in differentiating cochlear versus neural lesion sites can be limited.

Figure 6.4 Distortion-product otoacoustic emissions (DPOAE) of a normal-hearing patient (A) and a patient with sensorineural hearing loss above 2,000 Hz (B). (F2=second [higher] frequency.)

AUDITORY BRAIN STEM RESPONSE

The auditory-evoked potential (AEP) consists of a series of neuroelectric responses generated throughout the auditory pathway. It is seen as a transient neuroelectric pattern that is time-locked to an auditory stimulus and superimposed on the larger electroencephalographic (EEG) waveform. Components of the AEP occur as late as 500 msec after stimulus onset. Classification of the AEP is not yet standardized, but its components are usually organized according to their site of generation and latency. For example, responses can be categorized as "fast" (1–10 msec), "middle" (8–50 msec), "slow" (50–300 msec), and "late" (300+ msec).

The AEP that has received the greatest clinical attention is the "fast" response, referred to as the *auditory brain stem response* (ABR). The adult ABR is composed of seven wave peaks occurring within the first 10 msec after stimulus onset. The wave peaks are designated as roman numerals I through VII in the order of their latency of occurrence.[21] The wave peaks are products of graded postsynaptic potentials and action potentials from different locations along the auditory nerve and brain stem. The latency from stimulus onset to the wave peaks (absolute latency) and latency from peak to peak (interpeak latency) represent axonal conduction time to and between generator sites, respectively.

The ABR of an infant is different from that of an adult. The waveform is usually limited to three wave peaks that correspond to the adult waves I, III, and V. Absolute and interpeak latencies are longer than adult values, and amplitudes of the wave peaks are markedly different. Variations between the infant and adult response are attributed to several factors related to peripheral and central maturation. These include myelination, cochlear development, middle-ear condition, synaptic efficiency, and synchrony of neuronal firing.[22] Adult values are normally reached between 12 and 18 months of age.

Measurement of the ABR response presents a problem akin to that of finding a needle in a haystack. Stimulus-related potentials, including the ABR, are extremely small in amplitude when compared to that of the spontaneous EEG and other nonauditory physiologic potentials. The instrumentation used is designed to extract the ABR by maximizing its signal and minimizing extraneous physiologic and external "noise." This is accomplished by the use of specific electrode arrays, differential preamplification, filtering, analog-to-digital conversion, and repeated sampling and summation of the neuroelectric activity that is time-locked to auditory stimulation.

Successful measurement of clear and reliable ABR waveforms requires the use of acoustic inputs that produce a high degree of neural synchrony. In this context, synchrony refers to the degree to which simultaneous neuroelectric responses occur across a population of neural fibers. The greater the neural synchrony, the larger the magnitude of the ABR and the greater the time relationship of the ABR components to the signal onset. The highest degree of neural synchrony is achieved with a click stimulus because of its short duration and fast rise time. The use of the click, however, limits the interpretive power of the ABR because it is a broadband sound. Thus, in an effort to achieve neural synchrony, frequency specificity is lost. With the click stimulus, neural synchrony is greatest at the basal region of the cochlea, and it is generally assumed that the ABR response to click stimuli is correlated to behavioral threshold in the high-frequency region of 1,000–4,000 Hz. Other inputs having greater frequency specificity can be used during testing and are discussed in the following sections.

Clinical application of the ABR can be categorized into three major areas: (1) evaluation of the neural integrity of the auditory nerve and brain stem, (2) estimation of hearing threshold, and (3) determination of site of peripheral pathology. ABR testing is of particular value when assessing an infant because the measure does not require a voluntary, behavioral response and is unaffected by patient state and level of consciousness. Clear waveforms do require, however, that the child be relaxed, quiet, and unmoving. Most children between the ages of 8 months to 5 years are sedated before testing, usually with chloral hydrate. Neonates and infants younger than 8 months of age can be tested while in a natural sleep state. This state can be encouraged through sleep deprivation and feeding before testing. Children older than 5 years of age and adults can be tested in an awake state, provided they can remain relaxed and unmoving during test runs.

Evaluation of Neural Integrity

The ABR test is the most powerful tool in the audiologic battery for the identification of tumors of the eighth nerve and brain stem. The measure is also

Figure 6.5 Auditory brain stem response obtained from the right ear of a 32-month-old female patient (acquired at 95 dB nHL).

useful in identifying vascular lesions and the effects of demyelinating diseases. Neurologic assessment is conducted by presenting click stimuli at a suprathreshold intensity level. Most examiners test at levels between 75 and 95 dB nHL. (Zero dB nHIL denotes average normal-hearing threshold for a click stimulus.) A normal ABR obtained from the right ear of a 32-month-old girl is shown in Figure 6.5. In normal patients, wave I is seen to occur between 1.4 and 2.0 msec after stimulus onset, with each successive wave occurring at intervals of approximately 1 msec. Waves I, III, and V are generally the most prominent wave peaks and are used to interpret test findings. Hearing loss can have a significant effect on the absolute latencies of the ABR wave components. Wave I can be delayed or missing, or, in cases of severe hearing loss, the entire response can be absent. Although absolute latencies can be prolonged, interpeak latencies are not affected by conductive or cochlear hearing loss.

The most useful interpretive measure in neurologic assessment is interpeak latency, specifically, I–V, I–III, and III–V latencies. A normal I–V latency is approximately 4.0 msec, whereas normal I–III and III–V latencies are approximately 2.0 msec. Standard deviations are generally between 0.1 and 0.2 msec. Interpeak latencies are considered abnormal and indicative of neurologic abnormality when their values are greater than 2 standard deviations beyond the normal mean. When wave I is absent, interpeak latencies cannot be calculated. In these cases, the absolute latency of wave V or the interaural latency difference of wave V can be used for interpretive purposes.

A second indicator of neurologic pathology is the partial or complete absence of wave peaks in patients who possess significant residual hearing. For example, in cases of eighth nerve or low brain stem lesions, all waves beyond wave I may be missing. For lesions affecting higher portions of the brain stem, waves I and III may be present with wave V absent.

Other measures that indicate neurologic involvement include abnormal V–I amplitude ratios, "noisy" or poorly formed waveforms, and abnormal wave V latency shifts with increases in stimulus repetition rate.

Threshold Estimation

Stimulus intensity has a predictable and measurable effect on the ABR waveform. As stimulus intensity is decreased, wave components decrease in amplitude and increase in latency. Wave V is the most robust wave component and remains detectable at levels as low as 10 dB nHL. Other waves disappear at higher levels. For this reason, wave V is used as the basis for threshold estimation.

The threshold estimation procedure consists of obtaining ABR waveforms at decreasing stimulus intensity levels until wave V is no longer discernible. Wave V increases in latency on an average of 0.3–0.4 msec per 10 dB decrease in stimulus intensity within the range of 90–20 dB nHL. The lowest level at which wave V is detectable is referred to as *ABR threshold*. The exact relationship between ABR and behavioral threshold varies across test centers. Generally, when using a click stimulus, ABR threshold is reached 10–20 dB above behavioral threshold in the 1,000- to 4,000-Hz frequency range. Threshold estimation results for the previously described 32–month-old girl (Figure 6.5) are shown in Figure 6.6. As can be seen, wave V decreases in amplitude and increases in latency as stimulus intensity is reduced from 95 to 25 dB nHL. Wave V is visible to 25 dB nHL, suggesting normal hearing sensitivity in the 1,000- to 4,000-Hz region. Bone-conducted click stimuli can also be used to determine sensorineural reserve and, when compared to air-conducted click responses, can provide information concerning site of lesion (see Figure 6.6).

A 500-Hz toneburst stimulus can be used to obtain low-frequency sensitivity data. With this stimulus, the ABR waveform usually appears as a single, relatively broad wave peak. Its threshold is generally reached 30–40 dB above behavioral threshold at 500 Hz. This measure is useful for estimating the degree of low-frequency residual hearing and, when used in conjunction with the click stimulus response, can provide an approximation of the audiometric configuration.

Determination of Site of Peripheral Pathology

By determining wave V latency across a range of stimulus intensities, a latency-intensity function (LIF) can be constructed. An LIF is a graphic plot that

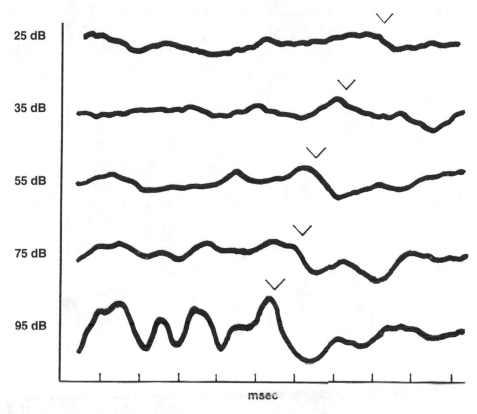

Figure 6.6 Threshold estimation results showing auditory brain stem response waveforms as a function of decreasing stimulus intensity.

shows wave V latency changes as a function of intensity. The LIF for the patient discussed above (see Figures 6.5 and 6.6) is shown in Figure 6.7. The unlined area represents the normal latency-intensity relationship. By plotting a particular patient's LIF and comparing its slope to that of normal results, information concerning site of pathology can be obtained. Cochlear losses often display a steeper LIF slope than normally seen. That is, wave V latencies increase at a faster rate with decreases in stimulus intensity when compared to noncochlear lesions and normal ears. Often, normal latencies are seen at high intensity levels. In conductive losses, the LIF is shifted to the right but demonstrates a slope similar to that seen for normal results (see Figure 6.7).

NEONATAL SCREENING

Optimal habilitation of the hearing-impaired requires identification of their disorder at the earliest possible time. Under ideal conditions, a congenitally hearing-impaired infant should be evaluated, fitted with hearing aids, and

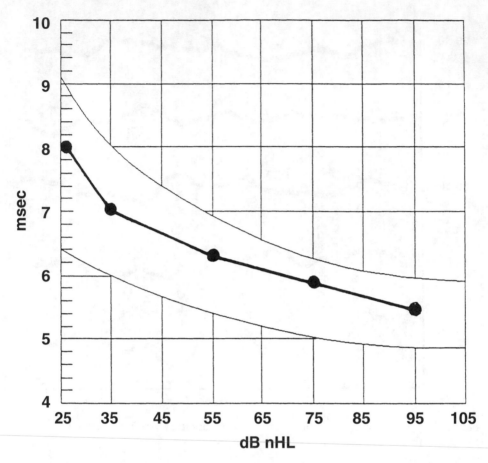

Figure 6.7 A wave V latency-intensity function. (Wave V latencies taken from Figure 6.6.)

enrolled in an aural habilitation program by 6 months of age. This requires the existence of effective and efficient neonatal screening programs and procedures.

The routine hearing screening of all newborns, referred to as *universal screening*, is the best way to identify children with hearing impairment at birth. Universal hearing screening has been endorsed by professional associations and infant-hearing task forces[15,23,24] and is in effect at many birthing facilities. For a significant number of centers, however, the cost of universal screening programs is prohibitive. In cases where universal screening is not possible, guidelines have been developed for the hearing screening of neonates and infants who are at risk for hearing impairment.[23,24] The risk factors apply to neonates (birth to 28 days) and to infants (29 days to 2 years) who develop particular health conditions that require (re)screening. Those children who manifest one or more of the risk factors should be referred for hearing screening. Although risk-factor screening is less costly than universal programs, it must be recognized that this approach identifies only 50% of children born with significant sensorineural hearing loss.[23,24] The risk factors included within the guidelines are as follows:

- A family history of hereditary childhood sensorineural hearing loss
- In utero infection (e.g., toxoplasmosis, other agents, rubella, cytomegalovirus, herpes simplex [TORCH])
- Craniofacial anomalies, including those with morphologic abnormalities of the pinna and ear canal
- Birth weight less than 1,500 g (3.3 pounds)
- Hyperbilirubinemia at a serum level requiring exchange transfusion
- Ototoxic medications, including but not limited to the aminoglycosides used in multiple courses or in combination with loop diuretics
- Bacterial meningitis
- Apgar scores of 0–4 at 1 minute or 0–6 at 5 minutes
- Mechanical ventilation lasting 5 days or longer
- Stigmata or other findings associated with a syndrome that is known to include a sensorineural or conductive hearing loss
- Parent or caregiver concern regarding hearing or developmental delay
- Head trauma associated with loss of consciousness or skull fracture
- Recurrent or persistent otitis media with effusion for at least 3 months

Some children are at risk for fluctuating, delayed-onset, or progressive hearing loss. In such cases, hearing should be monitored at least once every 6 months until 3 years of age, even if the child passes the initial screening. The risk factors for these types of hearing loss include the following[23,24]:

- Family history of hereditary childhood hearing loss
- In utero infection
- Neurofibromatosis type II and neurodegenerative disorders
- Recurrent or persistent otitis media with effusion
- Anatomic deformities and other disorders that effect eustachian tube function

Test procedures are identical for universal and risk-factor screening programs. Neonates should undergo hearing screening before being discharged from the hospital. The procedures of choice for neonates and infants up to 6 months of age are EOAE or ABR. Most centers use one or the other test, although the National Institutes of Health (NIH)[15] recommends that both tests be used under certain conditions. Under the NIH protocol, the use of EOAEs alone is sufficient if the screening is passed; if it is failed, it should be followed by ABR screening. This two-stage procedure is recommended because EOAE is a more rapid and cost-effective test but lacks the degree of specificity of the ABR test.

The pass criteria for EOAEs is the presence of emissions bilaterally at an acceptable signal-to-noise ratio in response to suprathreshold clicks in TEOAE screening or in response to a series of suprathreshold primary tones in DPOAE screening. The pass criterion for ABR is the presence of wave V bilaterally in response to click stimuli presented at 35 dB nHL or lower.[24]

For children between the ages of 6 months and 3 years, behavioral screening techniques can be used. VRA is the procedure of choice for children between the ages of 6 months to 2 years. Conditioned play audiometry can be attempted when screening the 2–3 year old. The pass criteria for these techniques are reliable responses to 1,000, 2,000, and 4,000 Hz pure tones presented bilaterally at 30 dB HL for VRA and at 20 dB HL for conditioned play audiometry. In cases where soundfield testing is necessary because earphone placement is not possible, parents should be advised that the existence of unilateral hearing impairment is not ruled out.[24]

Screening failures should be referred for audiologic evaluation to include behavioral testing, additional electrophysiologic testing, and immittance measures. Follow-up and management systems for children identified as hearing-impaired should include medical, otologic, and diagnostic and habilitative audiologic services.

REFERENCES

1. Northern JL, Downs MP. Hearing in Children (4th ed). Baltimore: Williams & Wilkins, 1991;139.
2. Bench J, Collyer D, Mentz L, et al. Studies in behavioral audiometry, III: six-month-old infants. Audiology 1977;15:384.
3. Eisenberg RB. Auditory Competence in Early Life. Baltimore: University Park Press, 1976.
4. Bench J. The law of initial value: a neglected source of variance in infant audiometry. Int Audiol 1970;9:314.
5. Liden G, Kankkunen A. Visual reinforcement audiometry. Acta Otolaryngol 1969;67:281.
6. Haug O, Baccaro P, Guilford F. A pure-tone audiogram on the infant: the PIWI technique. Arch Otolaryngol 1967;86:435.
7. Carhart R. Observations on relations between thresholds for pure tones and for speech. J Speech Hear Disord 1971;36:476.
8. Elliot L, Katz D. Development of a New Children's Test of Speech Discrimination. St. Louis: Auditec, 1980.
9. Erber NP. Use of the auditory numbers test to evaluate speech perception abilities of hearing-impaired children. J Speech Hear Disord 1980;45:527.
10. Jerger S, Lewis S, Hawkins J, et al. Pediatric speech intelligibility test, I: generation of test materials. Int J Pediatr Otorhinolaryngol 1980;2:217.
11. Ross M, Lerman J. A picture identification test for hearing-impaired children. J Speech Hear Res 1970;92:311.
12. Jerger J. Clinical experience with impedance audiometry. Arch Otolaryngol 1970;92:311.
13. Paradise JL, Smith C, Bluestone CD. Tympanometric detection of middle ear effusion in infants and young children. Pediatrics 1976;58:198.
14. Kemp DT. Stimulated acoustic emission from within the human auditory system. J Acoust Soc Am 1978;64:1386.
15. National Institutes of Health Consensus Statement. Early Identification of Hearing Impairment in Infants and Young Children. Bethesda, MD: National Institutes of Health, 1993;11.

16. Bray P, Kemp DT. An advanced cochlear echo technique suitable for infant screening. Br J Audiol 1987;21:191.
17. Norton SJ. Applications of transient evoked otoacoustic emissions to pediatric populations. Ear Hear 1993;14:64.
18. Prieve BA, Gorga MP, Neely ST. Otoacoustic emissions in an adult with severe hearing loss. J Speech Hear Res 1991;34:379.
19. Kemp DT. Evidence of mechanical non-linearity and frequency selective wave amplification in the cochlea. Arch Otorhinolaryngol 1979;244:37.
20. Lonsbury-Martin BL, McCoy MJ, Whitehead ML, Martin GK. Clinical testing of distortion-product otoacoustic emissions. Ear Hear 1993;14:11.
21. Jewett DL, Williston JS. Auditory-evoked far fields averaged from the scalp of humans. Brain 1971;94:681.
22. Cox LC. Infant Assessment: Developmental and Age-Related Considerations. In JT Jacobson (ed), The Auditory Brainstem Response. San Diego: College-Hill Press, 1985;297.
23. Joint Committee on Infant Hearing. 1994 position statement. ASHA 1994;36:38.
24. Audiologic Assessment Panel. ASHA Desk Reference. Rockville, MD: American Speech-Language-Hearing Association, 1997.

7

Assessment: Examination, Interpretation, and Reporting

Frances P. Billeaud

IDENTIFICATION OF ATYPICAL COMMUNICATIVE DEVELOPMENT

Communicative *forms* and *means* among very young children can be plentiful in the absence of severe disabling conditions or quite limited in the presence of such conditions. In typically developing children, acquisition of communicative skills progresses along a reasonably predictable path, and specific components of communicative competence are commonly measured by comparing a given child's status with sequences typically expected for the child's developmental age. For many children, however, individual circumstances require more intensive efforts to identify whether there is a problem with communicative development and, if a problem is present, to describe its nature, determine an appropriate treatment plan, and interpret the findings and recommendations to the child's family. This process can be undertaken either under a traditional clinical format or, usually more productively, with full participation of family members in each phase of the assessment.

Earlier chapters have explored the many possible causes and risk factors for compromised or atypical communicative development (see Chapters 1, 2, 3, and 5). Significant communicative delays or disorders require specialized investigation by professionals experienced in working with infants and toddlers.

The basic elements of conducting such an investigation are as follows:

1. The speech-language pathologist's (SLP's) knowledge of normal developmental patterns across modalities, against which a particular child's communicative development can be compared
2. The SLP's knowledge of factors known to cause or be associated with atypical development that may apply to a particular child
3. A complete history of the child's prenatal course, birth, and subsequent development through which clues to the child's condition can be obtained
4. Information provided by the parents about the child's development and communicative abilities

123

5. Examination of the oral mechanism, communication patterns, and related physical characteristics
6. Serial observation and analysis of the child's interactions with familiar caregivers and others
7. Play assessment

Using these seven approaches in combination, professionals are able to determine which children are at risk for or are already demonstrating atypical communicative development. There are, of course, tools that can assist the practitioner in conducting infant and toddler assessments. These are discussed in a later section of this chapter (see Communication Assessment Tools below). Each of the seven assessment elements is essential to arrive at a valid profile of a child with suspected communicative development problems.

The Triage Concept in Assessment

The task that is before the professional at this point in the assessment process can be considered a triage process similar to the three-level process described by Lewis and Fox.[1] Usually, it is possible to place communicatively at-risk infants and toddlers in one of three distinct groups by the end of the assessment process:

1. Children who have obvious handicapping conditions that have predictable effects on communicative development and that may (or may not) require consideration of alternative or augmentative communication
2. Children who can be identified as being at medical or biological risk for conditions that affect communicative development and for whom periodic monitoring or specific interventions are appropriate
3. Children who are at risk because of environmental factors that are known to affect communicative development and for whom other interventions, especially modification of the environment or of interactions with significant adults, are appropriate

This categorization is important to families and may determine access to services that their children may require or benefit from. Policies that govern services provided by a given agency or institution often affect the specification of treatment groups (see Chapter 1 for detailed discussion), making the triage concept useful.

The triage concept is not perfect. There are many factors that affect a child's development. Further, transactional processes *among* those factors can be more important than a given set of specific conditions in and of themselves. For example, a very low birth weight (VLBW) child with significant impairment, born to a family with little education and low socioeconomic status (SES), is at far greater risk than other VLBW infants who are physically resilient and are discharged to situations where ongoing medical care and appropriate stimulation are available. In fact, when biologically at-risk infants have access to early and ongoing medical care and appropriate environmental stimulation, some studies indicate that even those VLBW babies who experience respiratory distress syndrome and intraventricular hemorrhage can be expected to have typical communicative development "as long as there are no long-lasting health problems that follow from this experience" (p. 193).[2] A word of caution, however, must also be included: There are infants for whom tolerance for seemingly insignificant or marginal physical insults or environmental factors is so low that a single factor in and of itself is the critical element that affects subsequent development.[3]

With reference to low birth weight babies, Sherman and Shulman[4] stated, "[t]he presence of short-term effects does not necessarily mean that there will be long-term effects, and, conversely, just because no short-term effects are evident does not mean there will be no long-term effects" (p. 83).

Family Assessment

As SLPs undertake the task of assessing the child, it must also be acknowledged that the "history" of the child and family are constantly "under construction" with the passage of time and experiences of life. It is impossible to separate the experience of the child from the experience of the entire family. It is essential to understand the basic dynamics of the child's family to provide effective guidance and engage the family in effective planning and habilitation efforts that fit their individual circumstances. If the family grants permission, Part H/Part C require that a family assessment be completed and that such an assessment be family directed. Balancing the timing of the family assessment with the requirements of obtaining other information essential to the process of identifying parameters of the child's developmental problem(s) is an issue for the practitioner and the family to work out together. Dictates of reimbursement schedules, constraints of time within the professional's practice setting, and the family's ability to make time for (and possibly bear the cost of) additional visits are factors in arriving at the appropriate time to undertake this facet of the assessment process.

A tool to facilitate the family assessment, the eco-map, is described in Chapter 4 (see Chapter 4, Figure 4.1). Completion of the eco-map can be done in less than 1 hour. Another approach is to explain what it is, how it is used, begin the process of completing the instrument, and then send the parents home with the form to be completed at their leisure and before the next appointment. That method allows the parents more time to contemplate the many factors they deem important in their family dynamics and elements with which they deal from day to day. That approach adds to their perception that the practitioner truly believes that they are the experts on their own family.

Each child and family present a unique set of circumstances with which the practitioner must deal. The case history is indispensable for those who work with the infant and toddler population. The eco-map can be considered part of the case history.

Information Provided by the Parents About the Child's Communicative Abilities

Parental concerns are acknowledged by most professionals to be a valid screening tool. Even the two-question Parents' Evaluations of Developmental

Status,[5] which takes less than 3 minutes to complete, is reliable in correctly identifying at least 73% of children who are later diagnosed with communicative disorders through speech and language testing.[6] The two questions included on the questionnaire are (1) "Please tell me any concerns about how your child is learning, developing, and behaving" and (2) "Do you have any concerns about how he or she understands what you say? . . . talks? . . . makes speech sounds? . . . uses hands and fingers to do things? . . . uses arms and legs? . . . behaves? . . . gets along with others? . . . is learning to do things for himself or herself? . . . is learning preschool and school skills?"

As the SLP and parents engage in exchanges of information relating to the child's personal history, information is likely to be provided that opens the discussion to parental interactions with the child. Such interactions are generally not viewed as "communication encounters" by the parents, especially if the child is in a preintentional or preverbal developmental stage. Such discussions provide optimal opportunities for the SLP to discuss communicative means (e.g., eye-gaze shifts, gestures, facial expressions, vocalizations) and communicative functions. The examiner can then provide a list of functions appropriate to the child's estimated developmental level. The emergence of communicative intent can be determined and, if necessary, pointed out to the family as a step in the sequence of communicative development. A list of some of the more popular and useful parent questionnaires is provided in Table 7.1.

Table 7.1 Questionnaires Intended for or Adaptable to Parent Use in Determining Levels of Communicative Development in Infants and Toddlers

Questionnaire	Age	Reference
Denver Developmental Screening Questionnaire	0–6 yrs	31
Infant/Child Monitoring Questionnaire of Assessment, Evaluation, and Programming System	4–36 mos	32
MacArthur Communicative Development Inventory Infant Form and Toddler Form	10 mos–3 yrs	33
Language Development Survey	2 yrs	34
Parent Form: The Rosetti Infant-Toddler Language Scale	0–3 yrs	35
Cue Questions (intended for use with children who have developmental disabilities)	Adaptable to infants and toddlers	36
Receptive-Expressive Emergent Language Scale–2 (REEL-2)	1 mo–3 yrs	37
Semantic/Pragmatic Communication Report Form	Symbolic stages	38

The family and other caregivers are invaluable sources of information about what the child has done and is currently doing. Because parents know the child best and have observed and interacted with the child across time and across experiences, they are the experts on that child. Professionals need to affirm that fact in interactions with the family.

Examination of the Oral Mechanism, Communication Patterns, and Related Physical Characteristics

The oral mechanism is inspected for integrity of structure and function in the usual manner. The examiner also notes symmetry of facial features at rest and during movements. Although a baby is unlikely to follow the directive "pucker your lips," it is quite likely that the infant will mimic the examiner or parent's model of that movement to allow observation of motor function during the act.

Communication patterns of very young children can be described. Early interactions in which turn talking occurs can be observed. The child's ability to localize to sounds and voices, affective responses to the adult's tone of voice and loudness level, and development of intentional communicative acts to attract the attention of others or to engage in vocal play are also available for description.

The child's spontaneous vocalizations (e.g., coos, cries, babbling) can be used to assess characteristics of phonation (i.e., quality, pitch, loudness). Resonance characteristics are more easily detected in toddlers, but hypernasality and hyponasality can be discernible in babbling patterns of older infants If either is noted, further investigation of the cause is warranted. Assessment of respiratory function for vocalization (and verbalization in older babies) is also rated by the examiner.

Articulatory function is also assessed as soon as it is possible to do so. Variety in babbling is expected to emerge in predictable patterns with random sound production preceding reduplicative and canonical babbling. The phonemes of the language of the home gradually emerge as the preferred sounds for babbling. A method for analyzing infants' babbling patterns is outlined by Mitchell.[7] Such detailed analysis is not necessary if the SLP determines that babbling patterns are within expectations for the child's developmental age; however, the method described by Mitchell is useful when that is not the case. Children who do not exhibit variety in their babbling or whose babbling is discontinued after what appeared to be normal onset should alert the examiner to the possibility of a hearing impairment or other problem that results in delayed or disordered expressive language and speech at a later time.

As spoken words emerge, it is possible to determine the child's phonemic inventory for consonant and vowel production. Wetherby[8] suggested that production of different phonemes should approximate the following sequences for the ages shown: 8–12 months (prelinguistic stage), average of three; 12–15 months (early one-word stage), average of five; 15–18 months (late one-word stage), average of seven; and 18–24 months (multiword stage), average of twelve.

Physical characteristics to be observed include those that have their origins early in fetal development. These characteristics are sometimes referred to as *soft neurologic signs*, for they can be associated with some syndromes or conditions that are known to be related to communication difficulties. Bell[9] and Superneau[10] suggested making special note of the following traits, especially if they occur in combination:

- Head circumference out of the normal range on growth charts
- More than one hair whorl (cowlick) (Consider whether this is a family trait.)
- Very fine, electric hair
- Epicanthus
- Upslanted palpebral fissures in individuals not of Asian descent (less than 1% occurrence)
- Downslanted palpebral fissures (less than 1% occurrence)
- Hypertelorism (widely spaced eyes) (Beware of mislabeling this feature.)
- Malformed ears, absent ear lobe, microtia, atresia, skin tags
- Low-set ears (Be certain that you are not observing slight posteriorly rotated, rather than low-set ears.)
- High-steepled palate
- Furrowed or "geographic" tongue
- Curved fifth finger
- Single palmar crease (Palm creases are laid down at 12–14 weeks' gestation.)
- Webbing (syndactyly) of the fingers or toes
- Third toe longer than the second
- Splotchy pigment of the skin
- Absent or malformed fingernails and toenails
- Café-au-lait spots, which can be associated with neurofibromatosis

Bell[9] asserted that

as early as the first year of life there is an indication that infants with a high count of minor physical anomalies are not processing information properly, either having difficulty forming a schema from what is presented to them or forming a hurried, imperfect schema. They appear to shift from ponderous attention to flitting when they become fatigued (p. 29).

Such behavior has serious implications regarding communicative development, especially language development, which relies heavily on the child's ability to focus and maintain attention.

Superneau[10] reiterated the caution that diagnosis of syndromes and medical conditions should be matters entrusted to experienced physicians. Suspected problems should be referred; and families should be counseled by experts in the field.

Serial Observation and Analysis of the Child's Interactions with Familiar Caregivers and Others

Infants and toddlers are unique in that their endurance, attentiveness, and interests vary considerably with their caregiving requirements and routines, sleep and wake cycles, their sensitivity to new situations and people (e.g., the examiners), their attachment to the accompanying adult, and other factors that are not necessarily applicable to older children who have developed more mature patterns of behaviors and activities. It is crucial that practitioners who work with infants and toddlers have several opportunities to observe them and assess their behaviors and interactions rather than drawing conclusions based on observations obtained at a single visit. The potential for accumulating incomplete behavioral data leading to unfounded conclusions or misdiagnosis is high with this population.

To the extent possible, it is also imperative that the assessment of very young children be conducted in settings the children are accustomed to and in the company of familiar people—family members or regular caregivers. The dual evaluation tasks of the team or individual practitioner are "shopping for skills" (p. 65)[11] and identifying impediments to acquisition of communicative skills. It would be ideal if it were possible in every case to identify the source of the communicative delay or disability and to provide curative treatments. Unfortunately, that is seldom the final outcome of the assessment process because of the complexities of the variables involved and of their interrelationships.

Serial assessments of young children should include observation of their behaviors during routine daily activities, interactions with familiar people, manipulation of objects, and development of play. Videotaping the activities is highly recommended, as it frees the professional from the immediate need to document observations with paper and pencil and enables participation in—or at least undistracted observation of—the activity in progress. The videotapes can then be used to verify observed behaviors, detail or quantify the occurrence of specific communicative events, illustrate observations to the parent(s) by replaying pertinent sections of the tape, and contrast communicative behaviors in serial situations. Videotapes are also invaluable in tracking development and documenting acquisition of skills that were either absent or just emerging at the time of a given taping.

Novel situations should also be introduced during the serial assessment process. Wetherby and Prizant[12] provided suggestions that entice children to communicate during such encounters (see Appendix B for an adapted list of communicative temptations). In a sense, the assessment process can also be used as a "trial intervention" strategy. The child's responses to natural and novel bids for communication on the part of the parent or of the examiner in connection with ongoing activities that capture the child's attention for the moment may yield information about the child's preferred communication modes. Videotaped samples of the child's responses to specific strategies could be used later as a part of the parent-education program. It is obvious that this procedure has a direct bearing on assessment of play activities because play is the tool used to elicit the child's behaviors. Just as the sequence of communication development is generally predictable, so too is the sequence of play development.[13,14]

Atypical Child Behaviors

Children with delayed or disordered communication often use a variety of other, sometimes inappropriate, behaviors to express their needs and feelings. Persistence of problematic behaviors over time is a cause for concern, because they can interfere with social and even cognitive development. Observation of the child in the home, daycare setting, or professional's waiting room can yield significant information about apparent motivation to use vocal, nonverbal, and verbal communication; the adults' reactions to the child's communicative attempts (or lack of attempts); and what forms of nonverbal behavior are typically used by the child.

If there are persistent problematic behaviors about which the family is concerned, a referral to a mental-health professional may be indicated. Although there are no fixed guidelines for such referrals, Droter and Sturm[15] suggested referral if (1) the child's aggressive behavior interferes with the capacity to negotiate developmental tasks to the level of his or her assessed mental age or cognitive development; (2) the child's behavior interferes with responsiveness to early intervention services; or (3) the child's parents indicate that they feel high levels of stress about the child's psychological or interpersonal functioning.

Predictors of Language Development

As McCatherine and colleagues[16] pointed out, there are

four variables that appear to be closely related to language development and that independently predict language development irrespective of the presence or absence of other factors. . . . This small set of predictors includes three communication components that emerge during the prelinguistic period: (1) babbling, (2) development of pragmatic functions, and (3) vocabulary comprehension. The fourth predictor is the development of combinatorial and symbolic play skills (p. 58).

This set of four variables is expanded somewhat in terms of the pragmatic functions (see observations by Wetherby and Prizant in Four Groups of Concern to the Speech-Language Pathologist).

Traditional Assessment and Arena-Assessment Formats

Descriptions of multidisciplinary teams and their interactions are provided in Chapter 4. In their professional training programs, most practitioners in communicative disorders have been taught to assume significant, if not exclusive, responsibility for the communicative diagnostic or assessment process. The concept that individual SLP practitioners are legally and ethically responsible for their actions requires mastery of clinical skills in diagnosis, evaluation, and assessment. It is alarming to note that less than half of the graduates of programs in communication disorders have had exposure to the infant-toddler population. Over one-fourth of the respondents to a survey conducted by Dunn and colleagues[17] indicated that they "had no training with the birth-to-three population prior to graduation (not even units within a course); [only] 40% had an entire course" (p. 57). It is imperative that training programs provide students with opportunities to receive appropriate training with this age group.

Few training programs have implemented curriculum components that teach multidisciplinary or transdisciplinary team assessments, and even fewer provide training in arena assessment. Time constraints and competing priorities for curricular attention will probably continue to contribute to this dilemma. Fortunately, there is a considerable body of professional literature emerging on this subject, and increasing numbers of continuing-education programs are addressing these critical issues.

Although traditional clinical assessment methodology is essential, it appears that requirements of managed health care systems increasingly demand that practitioners also possess skills in team-assessment methodology, including arena assessment. Arena assessment is used when it is advantageous for one professional to handle the infant or young child while others look on. Planning of the assessment, including information desired by each participating professional, is completed either by the multidisciplinary professional team or by the parent(s) in conjunction with the professional team. A specialist in motor development is often designated to handle the child during the assessment so that muscle tone, reflex, and movement patterns can be judged. The entire multidisciplinary team, including the parents, participate in the process, exchanging information and providing each other with interpretations based on their individual areas of expertise. The process is different from either the solo evaluation or the traditional multidisciplinary assessment, both of which allow all participants direct access to the child.

Some emerging research is being directed at the arena-assessment issue and is also taking into consideration the increasing availability of electronic technology. Smith[18] reported on a developmental assessment model employed by the New York State Office of Mental Retardation and Developmental Disabilities that used a televideo network. Such assessment techniques have become common practice in some areas of medical practice. Perhaps some of the difficulties of providing appropriate services to children in rural or remote areas can be resolved in the future with refinement of technology and adaptation of procedures to the needs of very young children.

Play Assessment

Children's play is a rich source of information for professionals who study child development. Like physical growth, communication, and motor development, the development of play proceeds in a sequential manner along a reasonably predictable continuum. Appendix A provides a synopsis of expectations of typically developing play associated with the child's advancing age. Through play, which by definition is *fun*, it is possible to observe how a child interacts with objects, the immediate environment, and play partners. Underlying abilities, such as joint attention, sustained attention, manner and form of manipulation of objects, bids for interaction in play activities, and other attributes, can be judged through skillful construction of opportunities to observe the child at play. Play is a window through which it is possible to have at least a rough estimate of a child's cognitive abilities (e.g., through observation of problem-solving attempts, satisfaction of curiosity), temperament (e.g., through observation of exploring objects and surroundings, responses to frustration or directed attention, endurance), receptive communication (e.g., through observation of responses to requests or directives), expressive communication (e.g., through observation of body language [facial expressions, gestures, eye gaze], vocal and verbal expressions), and socialization. The child's levels of play schemes are also informative in connection with development of symbolic representations (e.g., use of a stick in place of a spoon in a kitchen play scheme). Demonstrated understanding of such representational symbols in play helps the SLP understand what is potentially available to the child in the area of verbal symbols.

Linder provided an excellent format for using play as a means of communicative assessment within the framework of a more extensive multidisciplinary assessment.[19] Resource references for using play as a foundation for assessment are provided in Appendix B.

INTERPRETING TO THE FAMILY

Sufficient time must be scheduled to provide information to parents. Depending on the family, the structure of the assessment itself, the setting(s) in which the assessment is conducted, and the amount of information to be shared, the interpretation may be provided at a single visit or may require two or more visits to complete. Parents may express a preference about the type and timing of the interpretation, designation of who should be present to hear the results, and where it would be most convenient to convene. The option of collaborating with families in that manner may be readily available to practitioners who work for agencies that are publicly supported and tend to be more permissive in terms of how much staff time can be expended in such endeavors. Certainly, best practices would be served under such circumstances. However, in light of the managed care environment in which many practitioners work, time may be more constrained; therefore, it may be necessary to condense the available information or to share it through written reports, followed by telephone consultations or brief office visits with a limited agenda relating to interpreting results of the assessment.

Although we may have logistical limitations imposed by administrative policy, SLPs must always keep in mind that they are talking to parents about their child: Emotions are inevitably involved and must be dealt with in an appropriate way. It is difficult for most professionals to deliver bad news when the outcome of the assessment is likely to be upsetting to the family; it is also difficult for the family to receive bad news. Sensibility and sensitivity demand best efforts to be both truthful and compassionate in providing information and its interpretation to families. Emphasizing what the child *can do* and *is doing* is both truthful and sensitive; providing information about what the next developmental level is likely to be is constructive; providing guidance to the family as to what they can do to facilitate movement from the present level of functioning to the next level is empowering and inspiring of hope—a valued commodity among parents of children with any kind of developmental delay or disability.

The process of assessment seeks to answer the following questions that parents and professionals have about a given child:

- What is happening here?
- What are this child's capabilities and limitations?
- What approaches can be used to promote the child's development?

The process of diagnosis seeks to answer the following questions:

- What is the accepted label for this condition or behavior?
- Why is this happening to this child?
- What is the etiology?
- What is the future course of development likely to be on the basis of historic documentation of other instances of the same condition or disorder?
- What are the appropriate treatment, intervention, and management options?
- What are the prospects for a positive outcome?

To arrive at the answers to these questions, other questions must be addressed. To prepare parents for a focused discussion at the meeting at which results of the assessment, diagnosis, and evaluation are shared, it may be helpful to provide the family with a list of questions each procedure endeavors to answer, so that at the time the family receives the interpretation there is a common ground for understanding what the professional(s) hoped would emerge from the evaluation. The assessment seeks to answer the following questions about the child's communicative status:

- What level of communicative development is expected of a child this age with the same or a similar physical diagnosis?
- What level of communicative development does this particular child exhibit?
- If there is a significant discrepancy, can the causes be established?
- What would constitute functional communication for this child?
- What abilities and strengths does the child possess through which other communicative skills can be developed?

- What are the forms and functions of the child's present communicative attempts?
- Who are the preferred communicative partners?
- What are the child's preferred settings for interactions?
- What are the barriers and limitations affecting communication for which compensation may be required?
- What needs to be done to assist this child to establish functional communicative competence?
- What are the family's priorities with respect to the use of assistive communication strategies or devices?
- What are the options for providing any assistance the child or family may need to achieve the desired outcome?
- How will progress toward the goals be evaluated?

FOUR GROUPS OF CONCERN TO THE SPEECH-LANGUAGE PATHOLOGIST

As SLPs consider how to classify the population of infants and toddlers they evaluate, it is useful to consider the general categorical groupings to which a given child may be assigned based on the outcome of the assessment process. Broadly speaking there are four such groups. Children in the first group have a diagnosed, handicapping condition that is certain to contribute to atypical communicative development. The second group is comprised of children who are established risk, and for whom it is highly probable that impaired communicative development will occur. Children in the third group are risk suspect; that is, biological, medical, or environmental conditions place them at a higher-than-average risk for future problems in developing communicative competence. Finally, there is a group with no known risk factor whose members, nevertheless, develop atypical communication.

For convenience, the groups are referred to as follows:

Group I: confirmed condition (+)
Group II: established risk (risk +)
Group III: risk suspect (risk ?)
Group IV: no known risk (risk 0)

A taxonomy for classifying children into the four groups is presented in Table 7.2.

Infants in group I are usually identified at or shortly after birth and begin early on to receive services from a variety of professional disciplines, although there are exceptions that tend to cluster in the last two categories listed under group I in Table 7.2.

Babies in group II may be identified at or shortly after birth but more often become the focus of concern when speech fails to emerge at the expected time (i.e., around 14–18 months of age or adjusted age if the baby was born preterm). Group-

Table 7.2 Suggested Taxonomy of Risk-Factor Groups Related to Communicative Impairment in Infants and Toddlers

Category	Examples of Specific Problems/Risks
Group I: Diagnosed conditions associated with atypical communicative development	
Sensory impairment	Hearing, vision, including retinopathy of prematurity, dual sensory impairment, and hyper- or hyporesponsivity to sensory stimuli
Physical conditions in which anatomic structures or neuromotor functions are impaired	Cerebral palsy, cleft palate, congenital craniofacial anomalies, intraventricular hemorrhage, bronchopulmonary dysplasia, laryngeal papillomatosis
Syndromes and genetic or chromosomal disorders associated with communicative disorders or mental retardation	Fragile X syndrome, Usher's syndrome, Down syndrome, Cornelia de Lange syndrome, Cruzon syndrome, cri du chat syndrome, Prader-Willi syndrome
Prenatal exposure to teratogens	Fetal alcohol syndrome, cocaine and other drug exposure
Diseases of newborns and infants in which known and unknown sequelae affect communicative development	Cytomegalovirus, human immunodeficiency virus, phenylketonuria, meningitis, rubella
Infant psychopathology (Note: Some problems can also be caused by genetic aberrations.)	Autism, pervasive developmental disorder, post-traumatic stress disorder
Problems of unknown etiology that are associated with impaired communicative development	Present with various, often multiple, disorders involving state regulation, neuromotor or sensory deficits, pervasive developmental delay, failure to thrive
Group II: Established risk: biological, medical, environmental risk factors associated with atypical communicative development	
Confirmed presence of family history for specific disorders	Learning disability, progressive hearing loss, language disability
Prenatal exposure to toxic substances without diagnosed sequelae at birth or during postpartum course	Cocaine, alcohol, prescription drugs (e.g., anticonvulsants)
Postpartum exposure to toxic substances	Antibiotic ototoxins, lead, neurotoxins
Prematurity and low birth weight, intrauterine growth retardation	<1,599 g <Tenth percentile in head circumference <37 weeks gestation Significant increase in risk if mother has little education and family is in a low SES group
Postmaturity	>40 weeks gestation (Note: Placental deterioration can be a factor in problems of postmaturity.)

Table 7.2 (continued)

Category	Examples of Specific Problems/Risks
Fetal distress or birth complications with or without diagnosed handicap at time of hospital discharge	Significantly prolonged labor, fetal distress, injuries from instruments
	Meconium aspiration, significant hypoxia or anoxia
Diseases and conditions	Rh incompatibility
	Apgar score lower than 7 at 5 mins
Atypical neuromotor or neurobehavioral function in infancy	Feeding or swallowing problems, hypersensitivity, inconsolability, hyposensitivity, floppiness, difficulty with state regulation, failure to thrive
Environmental	Very young mother in low socioeconomic status group with little or no formal education
	Strong family history of abuse or neglect
	Combination of such factors
Multifactorial	Early signs of possible developmental delay, attention deficit disorder, or learning disability

Group III: Risk suspect: conditions that suggest a significant risk of atypical communicative development
(Cumulative factors increase probability of atypical communicative development.)

Biological	Any inherent condition or combination of conditions that can interfere with normal neuromotor, physical, or sensory growth and development
	Soft neurologic signs
Medical	Any acquired disease, injury, condition, or combination thereof having the potential to interfere with normal neuromotor or physical growth and development or sensory integrity
Environmental	Any condition or combination of conditions having the potential to interfere with normal cognitive, social, psycho-emotional, communicative, or other developmental process

Group IV: No known risk factors in the presence of communicative delay or disorder
(Children in group IV can be reassigned to another group as maturation and discovery of applicable data lead to identification of previously unrecognized causative factors.)

II children often present clinically as being shy and exhibit meager social skills. However, some may present as aggressive children who are described as having behavior problems or suspected emotional problems. Their physical development and self-help skills may be age-appropriate, but their lack of ability to communicate verbally contributes to inappropriate use of other means of expression.[20]

The same is true of children in group III. As Wetherby and Prizant[21] observed,

> [s]ignificantly delayed referral is more likely to occur when no risk factors (e.g., very low birthweight, perinatal complications) have been identified or when communication and language delays do not coexist with significant physical, sensory, or cognitive disabilities, any of which may lead to earlier identification and more definitive diagnosis of developmental problems (p. 291).

Concern for development of these children may emerge at or about 14–18 months of age (adjusted age if the infant was premature) and may initially be centered on delayed onset of speech. However, if a child uses even a few words, parental concern may not emerge until considerably later: Age 24–36 months is not an uncommon referral point for such children. This is important to recognize because a substantial number of children between 24 and 30 months who have delayed expressive language, but whose receptive language skills are apparently intact, continue to exhibit expressive problems at ages 3 and 4 years.[22,23,24]

The SLP should be aware, however, that about half of children with intact receptive language at age 3 "catch up" with age peers in expressive language skills by the time of school entry. Parsing out which language-delayed children should receive treatment to optimize chances of normal language skills on school entry age is a challenge. Wetherby and Prizant[8] (p. 294) summarized the most pertinent indicators for persisting language problems in young children as follows:

- Deficits in the ability to share attention and affective states with eye gaze and facial expression
- A low rate of communicating with gestures and/or vocalizations
- A limited range of communicative functions, particularly lacking in the joint attention function
- A reliance on gestures and a limited use of vocalizations to communicate
- A limited consonant inventory and a less complex syllabic structure in vocal communication
- A delay in both language comprehension and production
- A delay in the spontaneous use of action schemes in symbolic play and the imitation of action schemes

These characteristics can be identified in children under the age of 18 months.

Concern for children in group IV may not develop until even later because some limited functional verbalization is almost always present early in life. Children who are initially considered to be group IV often escape notice until they reach the age of school entry, by which time standardized testing can be applied more reliably.

An interesting observation about children in group IV is that a significant number of them are observed to be "toe walkers." For reasons not yet clear, idiopathic toe walking (i.e., a diagnosis of exclusion in which diagnoses of spastic cerebral palsy, spinal dysraphism or injury, myopathy, neuropathy, autism, and pervasive developmental disorder [PDD] have been ruled out) seems to be a diagnostic sign of developmental language disorder (DLD). Accardo[25] and Schulman and colleagues[26] urged pediatricians to be aware of that phenomenon. Accardo stated, "[t]oe walking is a finding whose presence or history should strongly incline the clinician toward a neurologically based DLD" (p. 510). Schulman and colleagues, in their study of 799 children referred to an orthopedic clinic and seen by a multidisciplinary developmental evaluation team when toe walking was verified, observed that "[t]he [19] children in our study demonstrated delays in multiple developmental areas. Significant language delays were the most prevalent, occurring in more than 75% of the cases" (p. 545). They further commented that "an increase in the severity of language impairment was associated with an increase in the frequency of toe walking" (p. 545).

As noted throughout this book, value should be invested in the family's role in helping to identify children who are in need of communicative assessment. When parents are concerned about any aspect of their child's development, professionals should pay attention. Professional training programs usually include a study of the phenomenon of "parental denial" that can occur in the presence of identified problems, and instruction is provided on methods of dealing with it. Until recently, however, little attention was focused on the phenomenon of "professional denial," although parents have complained through the years about knowing something was wrong with their child and not being able to convince professionals to acknowledge the validity of their concern. Assurances by many professionals that the child would "outgrow" the problem were sometimes accurate but often represented a limited understanding of facts and resulted in delayed provision of appropriate care. When professional denial occurs, many months and sometimes years are lost to what might be appropriate preventive treatment or intervention during the optimal neurophysiologic developmental period.

ASSESSMENTS AND COMMUNICATIVE DIAGNOSES

Very young children who experienced professionals and parents place in one of the four risk groups defined above should have the benefit of a communication assessment or full communication diagnosis. Determining which of the two processes is appropriate at any point in time depends on individual circumstances, including the age and developmental status of the child for whom services are to be provided. Assessment is an ongoing process through which the child's present level of functioning is documented and strategies to enhance development and attainment of the next level of development are recommended. Many practitioners view the assessment process as part of developmental intervention activities. By contrast, as noted in Chapter 2 (see Screening, Evaluation, Diagnosis, and Assessment), the process of diagnosis has different goals and can be concluded with a referral to other personnel for habilitation or intervention services. Assessment of function is always a part of a diagnostic evaluation, but diagnosis is not necessarily a part of the assessment process. The two processes are intimately related but should not be considered interchangeable, although planning for both processes requires making decisions about what will be included in the process when it takes place.

As professionals consider the categories into which particular traits assign the child to diagnostic labels or functional descriptors, it is imperative that the implications of such labels and descriptors be considered.

Planning the Assessment

It may be useful to adopt a formal protocol for planning the process to be used. Adoption of such a planning protocol, which guides the sequence of activities and probably identifies personnel responsible for each step of the process, organizes the process for all participants and builds in a degree of predictability. It can also assist in developing projected timelines for the family and team of professionals involved. Table 7.3 illustrates what such a planning protocol can look like. The sequences can be modified to meet the needs of designated agencies or teams.

Communication Assessment Tools

Standardized Tests

Extreme caution should be exercised in using standardized tests with infants and toddlers. Careful consideration should be given to the norming population on which standardized scores are based: Potential exclusion from that group of children with the same diagnosed conditions as that of the child to be tested must make scores invalid. Extremely small samples or extremely varied conditions among children included in the normative group may make interpretation of individual scores extremely difficult. Very young children may not be able to comply with the protocol required in the prescribed testing procedures. Broad variations in developmental patterns among individual children can compromise reliability of test scores. Having said that, however, it must be recognized that in some states Part H/Part C service-eligibility regulations call for documentation of specific, quantifiable, deviations from the norm of standardized test scores. Hence, in some states, standardized testing is required to qualify children and families for early intervention services under Part H/Part C. Practitioners must be aware of such regulatory requirements.

Table 7.3 Suggested Sequence for Planning the Assessment

Receive
  Presenting concern or complaint
    Presented by whom (e.g., parent, other family member, professional[s], team)?
    What are the specifics of the concern or complaint?

Consider
  Validity of communicative concerns expressed in terms of risk groups shown in Table
    7.2 or other taxonomy

Evaluate
  Expressed or apparent need or rationale for service(s)
    Prevention (e.g., secondary, tertiary)?
    Scheduled monitoring (of developmental status, specific condition)?
    Evaluation? Assessment? Diagnosis?
    Statutory or regulatory compliance issues?
    Parent information, education, training?
    Habilitation?
    Rehabilitation?

Identify
  Protocol(s) to be employed and disciplines that need to participate
    Option 1: evaluation and assessment
      Neonatal intensive care unit assessment(s)
      Full developmental assessment
      Communicative assessment
    Option 2: diagnosis
      Comprehensive
      Communicative

Select
  Methods, tools, approaches to be used in developing the following:
    Case history
    Records review
    Observation of child and family
    Examination protocols: initial, serial
    Monodisciplinary, multidisciplinary settings
      Center
      Home
      Other site
      Combination of sites
    Approaches
      Multidisciplinary
      Transdisciplinary
      Interdisciplinary
      Arena format (standard or tele-electronic?)
      Consultation(s) needed
      Serial visit schedule (in consultation with family)
    Instruments, tools, procedures to be used

Conduct
  Assessment, evaluation, diagnostic examination(s)

Record
  Data generated by process used

Document
  Outcomes and impressions
  Evaluation and assessment of status
  Diagnosis
  Identified skills
  Strengths
  Needs
  Other findings

Prognosis (optional)
  For what?
    Development of functional communication?
    Development of oral communication skills?
    Development of age-appropriate oral communication?
    Other? (specify)

Determine
  What are the keys to a successful communicative and developmental outcome?
    Etiology and prognosis?
    Modifying identified perpetuating factors?
    Parent information, education, training, or any combination of these?
    Family involvement?
    Specific intervention, treatment, and management methods (e.g., assistive or augmentative communication)?
    Other means (e.g., referral for consideration of medical, surgical or other management)?

Recommend
  Treatment, management, and intervention plan
    Child-centered, traditional approach?
    Child-centered, family-focused approach? (Individual Family Services Plan)
    Other approach(es)? Special circumstances?
  Referral(s)
    For what?
    To whom?

Implement
  Intervention: treatment, management, or intervention plan
    Make appropriate referrals
    Recommend periodic re-evaluations if needed
    Implement active treatment, management, education
      Child
      Parents and family
      Other caregivers
    Monitoring and follow-up as recommended

Evaluate
  Outcomes
    Status
    Progress made since last visit or anticipated at next visit
    Need for modification of treatment or intervention plan

Judgment-Based Assessment

Judgment-based assessment (JBA) is a term used to describe the professional's authority, based on knowledge, training, experience, and status as a "qualified provider" under Part H/Part C, to determine a child's developmental status, strengths, and need for early intervention services. In some states, JBA is written into the assessment guidelines, having the effect of statutory authority invested in designated professionals to determine eligibility of infants and toddlers for Part H early-intervention services. Readers should note that regulations for PL 205-17, Part C (which becomes effective July 1, 1998), will become available after publication of this book.

Practitioners who apply JBA procedures use clinical-observation skills; devise situations in which the child's best "performance" can be expected or elicited; and integrate information from a wide range of sources to formulate an informed professional determination of the child's developmental status, observed strengths and needs, and recommendations for appropriate interventions. In some states, a combination of JBA and standardized testing is either required or permitted.

Initial concerns about a child's suspected atypical development are almost always based on JBA in the absence of known conditions or diseases present that are known to be associated with developmental disorders. As Morisset[27] observed,

> [e]ven though the range of normal variation in language acquisition is wide, there are robust indicators of potential difficulty, and these should not be ignored. Within the first year of life, early warning signs of language delay are apparent in the infant's lack of orientation to sound, social responsivity, or vocal play. By age 1, evaluation is warranted if a child is not using conventional gestures. Between 18 months and 2 years, indicators of potential delay are even more readily visible and include few spoken words, no comprehension of simple requests, or the absence of simple two-word phrases (p. vii).

Decisions that any one of those difficulties is present rest on JBA. Confirmation by formal testing may or may not be required under regulatory guidelines in the family's state of residence.

Multiple Strategies

Multiple strategies are required to develop an accurate picture of a child's communication system. Reliance on any one means or tool of assessment is to be avoided. The SLP employs both formally developed tools and JBA. Anecdotal reports can be as valuable to the assessment process as "hard data" (e.g., test results and physical measurements). The practitioner must be equally aware of available technology and equipment and of the ever-increasing number of tools and procedures that are being made available in contributions to the professional literature by commercial enterprise.

A number of formal diagnostic and assessment tools or instruments are available to practitioners. Some are standardized, some are criterion referenced (often to demonstrate attainment of specific skills or to generally accepted age norms for such attainment). Other tools are procedural strategies through which the child's behaviors can be analyzed with some degree of uniformity across populations. There are also questionnaires to be completed by parents or caregivers that are designed to elicit specific information about the child's developmental status, behavior, or specifics of health and treatments of record. Other tools deal with coping strategies used by parents, such as attitudinal scales by which it is possible to ascertain how designated individuals respond to the child or the disability or that identify family priorities with respect to enhancing parent's abilities to optimize their child's development.

Commercially available instruments vary widely in terms of (1) breadth of communication skills sampled, (2) depth of sampling, (3) methods of sampling used, (4) means of recording findings, (5) intended ages or conditions for which the instrument is applicable, and (6) criteria against which behaviors are compared. It is wise to be cautious in selection and application of instruments. This is doubly true when the child being assessed is known to possess sensory, cognitive, or motor impairments.

Qualitative and Multidimensional Scoring Systems

In some instances, consideration should be given to using a qualitative scoring system to document clinical observations. The child's mastery of a particular skill can be described as being present or absent, but it may also be valuable to describe the manner in which the child responds to specific stimuli. In this regard, examiners who are familiar with Porch's 16-point scoring system[28] or similar multidimensional systems may find them useful in conducting JBAs. Use of such systems is especially recommended in dealing with children who exhibit poor motor coordination.

Although such scoring systems do not yield standard, average, or mean scores, they are meaningful systems of describing skills or behaviors. Such systems, when used by groups of trained observers, also enable cross-validation of data for purposes of research and clinical application.

The Professional's Toolbox

Just as carpenters and plumbers need appropriate tools to fit a particular need, so does the SLP. To extend the analogy, master carpenters select among an array of hammers, saws, planes, and other tools the ones that will do a job most efficiently. In the same way, master plumbers rely on a variety of wrenches (e.g., monkey, crescent, ratchet, torque), knowing that different circumstances require different tools. Likewise, the SLP and other professionals who work with the infant-toddler-family population recognize the need for an array of tools that lend themselves to the requirements of specific situations.

A basic "toolbox" for the communicative disorders specialist may include the items listed in Table 7.4. Each practitioner discovers preferred instruments

Table 7.4 Selected Infant and Toddler Communication Assessment Tools

Instrument	Reference	Features	Recommended Age Group
Assessing Prelinguistic & Linguistic Behaviors	39	Observation and elicited interactions are used to assess cognitive antecedents to language, communicative intent, production and comprehension of language.	Birth to 2 yrs
Assessment of Mother-Infant Interaction	40	Observer rates mother-child interactions that are important to communicative development.	Birth to toddler
Assessment, Evaluation, and Programming System	32	It is designed as an interdisciplinary tool, but the "Social-Communication" section can be used separately by speech-language pathologists.	Birth to 3 yrs
Communication and Symbolic Behavior Scales (CSBS)	12	CSBS is a normed measure of communicative means, reciprocity, and social and affective signaling based on play activities and interactions with objects. (Note: Procedures can be adapted for less-structured evaluations for which norms do not apply.)	8 mos–2 yrs
Communicative Development Inventory for Infants	33	Inventory relies on parent reports of child's knowledge and use of prelinguistic skills and early language.	10–36 mos
Communicative Development Inventory for Toddlers	33	Inventory relies on parent reports of child's understanding and use of early language components.	10 mos–3 yrs

Instrument	Reference	Features	Recommended Age Group
		Recommended for children who have begun to use single words or connected speech.	
Cue Questions	36 (See Appendix B, Table B.2)	It is a parent questionnaire that gathers information on communicative means and functions of multiply handicapped or severely delayed children who function at levels expected of infants and toddlers. Checklist ranges from preverbal and nonverbal to phrase and sentence level.	Any, but nicely adapted to situations in which time constraints are present
Integrated Developmental Experiences Assessment (IDEAS)	41	IDEAS is a functional-language assessment based on observation of cognitive, social, and communicative behaviors in naturalistic settings. The focus is on integration of functions.	Birth to 36 mos
The Language Development Survey	34	It is a parent questionnaire that documents language usage of 2 year olds. It can be administered as a paper-and-pencil task or by interview.	2 yrs only
Preschool Language Scale–3	42	This standardized tool evaluates auditory comprehension, articulation, grammatical form and structure, and basic concepts of toddlers. It requires focused attention of the child to respond to picture prompts and listen to oral directions.	Toddlers

Table 7.4 (continued)

Instrument	Reference	Features	Recommended Age Group
The Rossetti Infant-Toddler Language Development Scale	35	It is a parent questionnaire and protocol for complete language assessment. It is criterion referenced. It uses observation, parent report, and elicitation of behaviors in play settings to generate data. The focus is broad and includes attention to attachment-interaction, pragmatics, gesture, play, preverbal communication, language expression, and comprehension.	Birth to 3 yrs
Transdisciplinary Play-Based Assessment	43	It is intended for use by transdisciplinary early intervention teams; however, the section on language assessment can be used by the speech-language pathologist alone. It provides an excellent overview of using play as a basis for assessing many facets of language development and use.	Developmental level of 6 mos–6 yrs

that meet the needs of a particular situation, practice setting, or both as new products and protocols are developed. The list provided in Table 7.4 reflects the author's selection of basic tools appropriate to a practice based in a university training program and its affiliated clinic. An expanded list of assessment tools is provided in Appendix B, Table B.1.

REPORTING RESULTS

Written reports are generally required and can be presented to the family at the time the results are interpreted to them by the professional team, its representative, or the individual practitioner. The format of written reports is often dictated by the agency, protocols of the practice group or practitioner, requirements of a funding agent, or other entity. Some written reports are lengthy (this is usually the case in clinical training programs); some are very brief (sometimes even to the point of being formatted as checklists or fill-in-the-blank forms); and others fall somewhere between those extremes. Reporting results to parents following the assessment or diagnostic process is discussed earlier in this chapter, see Interpreting to the Family. Written reports of professionals are generally considered to be eligible for subpoena in lawsuits as legal documents relating to the child's status.

Individual Family Service Plan

The individual family service plan (IFSP) is a unique requirement of Part H/Part C. It is viewed as both a process and a document that serves as a guide for intervention services selected by the family for their child or for the family itself as a means to enhance their ability to maximize the child's development. The IFSP is flexible, subject to change as the parents desire, and developed by the family in conjunction with members of the multidisciplinary team or the designated family services coordinator. By law, the IFSP must contain the following:[29,30]

- A statement of the child's present health status
- A statement of the child's developmental levels: physical (including sensory), cognitive, motor (gross and fine), communicative (speech and language), and social and emotional
- The service coordinator's name
- Expected outcomes (functional goals) for the child and family
- A listing of services to be provided
- Starting date and expected frequency and duration of the services and the person or agency responsible for providing the services
- Identification of the environment in which the services are to be provided (The child's normal environments [e.g., home, daycare center] are preferred and must be used to the extent possible.)
- A transition plan in anticipation of any major changes as the child moves from service to service or approaches the age of 36 months, at which time Part H/Part C services are terminated

In some instances, the IFSP can itself be regarded as the assessment report. Most agencies and practitioners, however, feel obligated by standards of practice to generate more specific written reports of assessment or diagnostic findings.

The family service coordinator is required to document how the IFSP services are to be financed. Payment through Part H/Part C funds in participating states is available only as a last resort; all other possible sources of payment must be tapped and exhausted before Part H/Part C funding can be requested. Some Part H/Part C services must be provided free of charge to eligible infants, toddlers, and their families. These include screening and evaluation, multidisciplinary assessment, medical services and equipment that are required to complete the multidisciplinary assessment, development of the IFSP, case management (service coordination), and transition planning.

Once an IFSP has been developed, the lead agency in the participating state is ultimately responsible for seeing that the designated services are provided through the family-focused, community-based system. Families can change the services that they request from time to time and can decline to participate in services for which they and the child are eligible. Any variation from the original IFSP requires a modification of that document. Families are entitled to initiate due-process proceedings when conflicts about services cannot be resolved with service providers. Eligibility criteria, policies relating to confidentiality and due process, and other components of a state's Part H/Part C implementation plan vary widely among participating states. Diagnostic and assessment processes can be affected by the rules and regulations pertaining to those aspects of the Part H/Part C system. Information about implementation is available from the state's lead agency. Lead agencies are listed in Appendix C, Table C.1.

Documentation must be made available by agencies and practitioners to designated monitors of the Part H/Part C system. Thus, assessment and diagnostic reports are essential records of the agencies and practitioners serving the Part H/Part C population.

Other Report Formats

Reports provided to other professionals can take the form of a personal letter or memo summarizing findings to which a more detailed report may be appended. Physicians and other professionals frequently prefer receiving one- (at most two-) page summaries of findings with a note that a more detailed report is available on request. In private practices and in managed health care environments, where time is a crucial element of the economic picture, economy of writing (and reading) time is at a premium. SLPs should cultivate skills in preparing information-dense but concise reports. However, there must also be a means of capturing the "fine-grained" information generated during the assessment or diagnostic process that leads to formulation of conclusions about a given child's communication system.

SUMMARY

Certain philosophical and procedural adaptations are required when different service-delivery models are used. Practitioners who serve the youngest segment of the pediatric population and their families need to keep abreast of rapidly developing legislative mandates, guidelines of practice, and technical advances through continuing professional education. The material presented in this chapter should confirm the reader's perception that mastery of specific technical skills, along with a healthy dose of common sense, go into the processes of assessment and diagnosis with very young children and their families, and that work with infants and toddlers is not simply a downward extension of skills applied with older preschool children.

Table 7.5 provides the reader with a condensed review of the necessary elements of a communication assessment.

Table 7.5 Quick Review of Items Essential to Communicative Assessment and Diagnosis

Review of records
   Medical and surgical
   Developmental
      Health status
      Physical and sensory development
      Cognitive development
      Motor development (i.e., gross and fine)
      Social-behavioral development (i.e., attachment, temperament, adjustment, coping behaviors)
      Communicative development (i.e., interactions, turn taking, means, intent, preverbal, receptive, expressive, nonverbal, verbal)
Pertinent history by interview
   Family (i.e., medical, social, and educational)
   Prenatal (child and mother)
   Postnatal
   Developmental
      Attainment of milestones
      Variations in development
      Problems and delays encountered
Presumed cause of present concern
   By family
   By professionals
Observation
   Child, parent, and family interactive styles
   In familiar and unfamiliar settings
   Videotaped record, if possible
Team participation[a]
   Family member(s)
   Speech-language pathologist
   Audiologist
   Psychologist
   Physician(s) (e.g., pediatrician, neurologist, ophthalmologist, orthopedist, radiologist, otorhinolaryngologist, gastroenterologist, plastic surgeon, geneticist, cardiologist, other specialist)
   Physical therapist
   Occupational therapist
   Nurse
   Social worker
   Early childhood educator, early interventionist, early childhood special educator, child development specialist
   Other(s)
Examination, assessment, and evaluation
   Evaluation of sensory integrity (especially hearing, taction, vision, balance, tolerance for sensory stimuli)
   Evaluation of anatomic structures required for communication, including the peripheral oral mechanism and related physical structures
   Evaluation of physiologic function required for communication

Table 7.5 (continued)

Documentation of known conditions and syndromes that are or may be associated
    with atypical communicative development
Assessment of feeding and swallowing functions, if needed
Identification of communicative means, modes, functions, and intent
Assessment of communication status[b]
    Presymbolic
    Nonverbal symbolic
    Verbal
The communication examination and assessment also includes evaluation of the following:
    Interaction between child and primary caregiver(s) and interactive styles of family unit
    Cultural milieu in regard to communicative development
    Motivation for communicative effort
    Opportunities presented for communication within daily routines
    Play behaviors (i.e., cognitive and motor abilities, social interactions,
        coping skills, and communication skills exhibited)
Decisions to be made
    What to cover in examination(s)
    When examination(s) will be conducted
    Where examination(s) will be conducted
    How examination(s) will be conducted
    What special methods and tools are needed
        Laboratory tests
        Developmental inventories
        Specific test materials, instruments, equipment
        Special handling (e.g., therapeutic positioning)
        Videotaping of all or portions of the examination (for baseline reference and later
           comparison? for verification of findings? to free up examiners from documenta-
           tion chores during the examination? for viewing by team members not available
           at scheduled examination appointment?)
        To what extent will judgment-based assessment be accepted as part of the findings?
        In what format will documentation and reports be developed and disseminated?
What permissions and informed consent documents are required, and whose
    responsibility are they?

[a]Part H/Part C regulations define the multidisciplinary team as having at least two professional
members. A minimal team considered appropriate to communication examination comprises par-
ent(s), the speech-language pathologist, and the audiologist.
[b]See Appendix A for helpful reference data.

REFERENCES

1. Lewis ML, Fox N. Issues in Infant Assessment. In CC Brown (ed), Childhood
   Prenatal Risk: Pediatric Round Table #9. Skillman, NJ: Johnson & Johnson
   Products, 1983;78.
2. Menyuk P, Liebergott JW, Schultz MC. Early Development in Full-Term and
   Premature Infants. Hillsdale, NJ: Erlbaum, 1995;193.

3. Keefe KA, Feldman HM, Holland AL. Lexical learning and language abilities in preschoolers with perinatal brain damage. J Speech Hear Disord 1989;54:395.
4. Sherman T, Shulman BB. Low birthweight and developmental delays: research issues in communication sciences and disorders. Contemp Issues Communication Science Disord 1997;24:79.
5. Glascoe FP, Altemeier WK, MacLean WE. The importance of parents' concerns about their child's development. Am J Dis Child 1989;143:855.
6. Glascoe FP. Parents' concerns about children's development: prescreening technique or screening test? Pediatrics 1997;99:522.
7. Mitchell PR. Prelinguistic vocal development: a clinical primer. Contemp Issues Communication Sci Disord 1997;24:87.
8. Wetherby AM. Alton Ochsner Clinic Annual Continuing Medical Education Program: Infants and Toddlers with Special Needs, New Orleans, May 1996.
9. Bell RQ. Minor Physical Anomalies: Relation to Later Achievement. In NW Paul (ed), Research in Infant Assessment. White Plains, NY: March of Dimes Birth Defects Foundation, 1989;25.
10. Superneau DW. Subtle Signs of Undiagnosed Genetic Disorders ("The Dysmorphology Detective"). Paper presented at Conference on the Child with Special Needs, New Orleans, April 1997.
11. LeVan RR. Clinical sampling in the assessment of young children with handicaps: shopping for skills. Top Early Child Special Educ 1990;10:65.
12. Wetherby AM, Prizant BM. Communication and Symbolic Behavior Scale [CSBS] – Normed Edition. Chicago: Applied Symbolix, 1993.
13. Fewell R. Play Assessment Scale. Miami: University of Miami, 1991.
14. Fewell R. Assessing the Child with Special Needs Using Play Observations: Evaluating Communication, Cognition, and Motor Behavior. Paper presented at the Conference on the Child with Special Needs, New Orleans, April 1997.
15. Droter D, Sturm L. Mental health intervention with infants and young children with behavioral and developmental problems. Infants Young Child 1991;3:1.
16. McCatherine RB, Warren SF, Yoder PJ. Prelinguistic predictors of later language development. In KN Cole, PS Dale, DJ Thal, Assessment of Communication and Language. Vol. 6: Communication and Language Intervention Series. Baltimore: Paul H. Brookes, 1996;57.
17. Dunn SL, van Kleeck A, Rossetti LM. Current roles and continuing needs of speech-language pathologists working in neonatal intensive care units. Am J Speech-Lang Pathol 1993;2:52.
18. Smith DL. Teleassessment: a model for team developmental assessment of high-risk infants using a televideo network. Infants Young Child 1997;9:58.
19. Linder TW. Transdisciplinary Play Based Assessment. Baltimore: Paul H. Brookes, 1993.
20. Prizant BM, Meyer EC. Socioemotional aspects of language and social communication disorders in young children. Am J Speech-Lang Pathol 1993;2:56.
21. Wetherby AM, Prizant BM. Toward Earlier Identification of Communication and Language Problems in Infants and Young Children. In SJ Meisels, E Fenichel (eds), New Visions for the Developmental Assessment of Infants and Young Children. Washington, DC: Zero to Three/National Center for Infants, Toddlers, and Families, 1996;289.
22. Rescorla L, Schwartz E. Outcome of Specific Language Delay (SELD). Paper presented at the meeting of the International Conference on Infant Studies, Washington, DC, April 1988.
23. Fischel J, Whithurst G, DeBaryshe B. Language growth in children with expressive language delay. Pediatrics 1989;83:218.
24. Rescorla L, Roberts J, Dahlsgaard K. Late talkers at 2: outcome at age 3. J Speech Hear Res 1997;40:556.

25. Accardo P. On one's toes about developmental language disorders. J Pediatr 1997;130:509.
26. Schulman LH, Sala DA, Chu MLY, et al. Developmental implications of idiopathic toe walking. J Pediatr 1997;130:541.
27. Morisset CE. Perspective. Infants Young Child 1997;9:vi.
28. Porch BE. Porch Index of Communicative Ability in Children. Palo Alto, CA: Consulting Psychologists Press, 1979.
29. Public Law 102-119. Amendments to the Individuals with Disabilities Education Act [IDEA] of 1991.
30. Public Law 205-17. Amendments to the Individuals with Disabilities Education Act (Part C) of 1997.
31. Frankenburg WK and Dodds. Denver Developmental Screening II. Denver: Ladoca Project and Publishing Foundation, 1990.
32. Bricker D. Assessment, Evaluation, and Programming System (AEPS) for Infants and Children, Vol 1: AEPS Measurement for Birth to Three Years. Baltimore: Paul H. Brookes, 1993.
33. Fenson L, Dale PS, Reznic JS, et al. MacArthur Communicative Development Inventories for Infants and Toddlers. San Diego: Singular, 1991.
34. Rescorla L. The language development survey: a screening tool for delayed language in toddlers. J Speech Hear Disord 1989;54:598–599.
35. Rossetti LM. The Rossetti Infant-Toddler Language Scale: A Measure of Communication and Interaction. East Moline, IL: LinguiSystems, 1990.
36. Schuler AL, Peck CA, Willard C, Theimer K. Assessment of communicative means and functions through interview: assessing the communicative capabilities of individuals with limited language. Semin Speech Lang 1989;10:51–62
37. Bzoch KR, League R. Receptive Expressive Emergent Language Scale (2nd ed). Austin, TX: PRO-ED, 1991.
38. Crais E. Communication Report Form. In DB Bailey Jr and M Wolery, Assessing Infants and Preschoolers with Handicaps (2nd ed). New York: Merrill, 1996;366–367.
39. Olswang L, Stoel-Gammon C, Coggins T, Carpenter R. Assessing Linguistic Behaviors. Seattle: University of Washington Press, 1987.
40. Klein MD, Briggs MH. Observation of Communicative Interaction. Los Angeles: Mother-Infant Communication Project, University of California at Los Angeles, 1987.
41. Norris JA. Assessment of Infants and Toddlers in Naturalistic Contexts. In WA Secord and JS Damico (eds), Best Practices in School Speech-Language Pathology: Descriptive/Nonstandard Language Assessment. San Antonio: The Psychological Corporation, 1992.
42. Zimmerman IL, Steiner VG, Pond P. Preschool Language Scale (3rd ed). San Antonio: The Psychological Corporation, 1992.
43. Dickson K, Linder TW, Hudson P. Observation of Communication and Language Development. In TW Linder, Transdisciplinary Play-Based Assessment. Baltimore: Paul H. Brookes, 1993.

8

Treatment, Management, Intervention: Optimizing Communication Development

Frances P. Billeaud

INDIVIDUALIZED CARE

Once it has been determined that a child needs developmental assistance, it is imperative that the assistance be appropriate to that child's needs. Brazelton[1] pointed out that oversimplified, nonindividualized intervention programs can do more harm than good. The individualization of intervention programs and attempts to help the young child acquire the power of functional communication are critical to creating optimal results. Individualized plans accentuate what the child *can already do* and what the parent-professional team can do to build on existing abilities. A positive and productive starting point is to identify the parents' priorities for the child. The professional's knowledge and technical expertise can then be used to assist in guiding family efforts to enhance the child's development. Goals can be modified over time, but the initial objectives that help the child progress from present status to the next developmental level provide a positive framework with a sense of purpose for all involved in the child's care.

IS IT TREATMENT, MANAGEMENT, OR INTERVENTION?

The terms *treatment*, *management*, and *intervention* have distinct meanings to practitioners in different work settings. For many, treatment implies a medical or allied-health approach to ameliorating or eliminating a diagnosed problem. Management, on the other hand, can subsume treatment but includes other processes through which a positive outcome is achieved. Management can include parent education, genetic counseling, and other measures not involving medication, direct therapeutic strategies, or surgical intervention. Treatment is often thought of as what is done to or for the individual possessing the diagnosed problem, whereas management usually involves parents, other caregivers,

153

and possibly program personnel. Intervention is designed to produce a favorable result for an identified problem. In the context of working with infants, toddlers, and their families, intervention has come to mean anything done that has a positive effect on enhancing the child's development. By contrast, intervention, as it is used in the field of mental health or substance abuse, implies a confrontation of the individual with the problem by loved ones, coworkers, or both to force the individual to face the seriousness of a situation and to initiate treatment. Because these terms are used in various ways by practitioners in different work settings, different disciplines, and the public, it is wise to ensure that professionals and family members understand what is meant when specific terms are used. The power of such terms to affect cooperation and involvement should never be underestimated.

Whatever the mechanism (management, treatment, or intervention) used, the same goal is operative: All efforts are directed by those involved to optimize the child's development. The speech-language pathologist's (SLP's) role in treating, managing, or intervening with the target population is multifaceted. Circumstances surrounding the child's care can be complicated or relatively straightforward. The activities in which the SLP engages are affected by philosophies of care, timing of treatment or intervention, the contributions of other professionals and caregivers to the processes, the child's condition and need for specific types of intervention, and other factors. Table 8.1 provides an overview of the many elements that must be considered.

STRATEGIES OF THE SPEECH-LANGUAGE PATHOLOGIST WITH THE PEDIATRIC POPULATION

Services provided by the SLP can include one or a combination of the following:

- Screening, referral, and follow-up
- Consultation
- Parent education
- Parent training
- Direct treatment and management of the delay or disorder
- Prevention
- Application of Part H/Part C intervention mandates

Screening, Referral, and Follow-Up

Parents or others may bring their concerns about the child's communicative development to the SLP through their own initiative or as a result of a referral from another parent or a professional. When the concern is reviewed by the SLP, it becomes apparent whether an immediate referral to another professional discipline or program is warranted or if the SLP should

Table 8.1 Treatment, Management, and Intervention Targets for Infants and Toddlers at Risk for Communicative Disorders

Child Centered	*Family Focused*	*Environment Focused*

For children with conditions that affect growth, structures, or functional integrity needed for communicative purposes
Single-discipline or multi-disciplinary management by the following:
    Medical practitioners in various specialties
    Surgical practitioners in various specialties
    Occupational therapist
    Physical therapists
    Nutritionist
    Audiologist
    Speech-language pathologist
    Psychologist
    Early childhood educator
    Specialists in prosthetic appliances and augmentative devices
    Case manager or service coordinator
	Parent training in techniques and methods specific to their child's physical and developmental needs
	Parent information and education about the following:
	    Decision making
	    Advocacy
	    Child development
	    Their child's condition or diagnosis
	    Financial resources
	    Legal rights of child and family
	    Available management options
	    Gaps in the service-delivery system
	    Family empowerment (identifying, selecting, and using services)
	    Self-advocacy
	    Service coordination
	    Family support for individual family members and the family unit as a whole
	    Social services
		Modifications (e.g., special equipment, furnishings, room arrangements, schedules) to enhance the child's development in various settings:
		    Hospital
		    Home
		    Center
		    Child care
		    Preschool
		    Clinic
		    Center

personally see the child to evaluate reported behaviors that may validate the need for concern or reassure the family that development is proceeding along a typical course. On the basis of these findings, the SLP can suggest a follow-up phone call or visit at some future date for the purpose of tracking the child's development.

Medical and surgical treatment may be warranted for some youngsters with delays or disorders in communicative development. Perhaps the most obvious problems for which surgical treatment would be appropriate are cleft lip, cleft palate, and other craniofacial anomalies. Surgical treatment can also be appropriate for certain laryngeal structural anomalies, granulomas, papillomatosis, and laryngeal trauma. Tracheotomies are required for a variety of problems. Pressure-equalization tubes are the treatment of choice for some chronic middle-ear infections. The role of the SLP in such instances can include referral to the medical practitioner on the basis of the quality of the child's vocalizations, parent reports of repeated earaches (especially if they have gone untreated), or physical characteristics that can be suggestive of a recognizable syndrome or are associated with motoric functioning of the oral mechanism.

The cost of referral service varies from one work setting to the next. Because the SLP's time is a commodity of the health care marketplace, a nominal fee may be charged. The service is one of the designated "free" services under Part H/Part C legislation, however, and many agencies absorb its cost as a function of public awareness and prevention activities.

Consultation

Consultation services are often provided in connection with care options considered or offered by other professionals (e.g., physicians, early interventionists, physical and occupational therapists). Such services are often part of the process for developing the individualized care plan. Consultation can be conducted as part of the discharge plan when an infant or young child is being released from a stay in the hospital, as part of an overall health care plan for a child with specific medical or surgical needs, or as part of the individual family services plan (IFSP) process when the multidisciplinary evaluation has been completed. When the service is provided as part of the development of the IFSP, it is free of charge to the family, and the agency can bill the Part H system directly for the allowable costs. When it is done as part of the planning process with peer professionals, the work setting generally dictates how the costs of providing the professionals' time are covered.

Coleman and colleagues[2] provided a perspective on the professional's role in serving as a consultant to parents. They observed that this form of consultation generally takes the form of (1) determining the nature of the problem at hand, (2) devising a plan to observe and record instances of the child's behavior that the family wishes to modify, and (3) helping the family to develop a plan of action to change the behavior to a desired outcome. They stated,

> [c]onsultee acceptance of the implementation plan and behavioral objectives is enhanced by . . . participation and input into the behavioral consultation process. Consultees are asked to contribute information on strategies that they have tried and on the level of success or failure of a particular strategy. . . . Most important, consultees assist in developing a plan of implementation that best suits their particular situation (p. 194).

They concluded, "[p]arents say that their major areas of need are for information and support, both of which consultation readily provides in a less intrusive format" (p. 198).

Formal and informal opportunities to provide in-service training and staff-development training are also forms of consultative services. If the medical staff is unfamiliar with the range of assistance the SLP can provide, a written communication or face-to-face meeting may be warranted. Seeking opportunities to address groups of specialists at their professional meetings is one way of conveying information about the SLP's technical competencies and desire to enhance the provision of comprehensive patient care. Providing copies (or abstracts) of pertinent articles from professional journals (both theirs and SLP journals) or reviews of pertinent new books, along with a short personal note to the appropriate medical staff members, is another way of breaking the ice with pediatric care providers; it is also a legitimate form of consultation.

Children who are under medical care for acute or chronic conditions can also benefit from what the SLP has to offer. Hospital pediatric care plans often reflect a concern for the child's lack of normal social stimulation and separation from family routines that are necessitated by periods of hospitalization. Staff communication with the child and with the family is a primary concern. The SLP can be of assistance in consulting with the medical and nursing staff about how to make the child's communicative stimulation as normal as possible under the circumstances. When children are under specific treatment protocols that require special equipment or pharmacologic management, the SLP can provide counseling with families about how to establish, strengthen, or optimize communication under such unusual circumstances. The SLP can also design temporary assistive communication strategies (e.g., basic communication boards for toddlers) and train the family and staff in their use.

Because development of communication skills occurs simultaneously with other aspects of child development, specialists can learn from one another. Sharing information about standard protocols of treatment, criteria for selecting or administering specific kinds of care, pertinent research findings, and how each member of the developmental team can assist the others in attaining their respective goals is an invaluable activity of the team. That type of consultation promotes a deeper understanding of the contributions of each discipline to optimal outcomes, enhances the skills of all team members, and improves the ability of members of the team to make appropriate referrals and provide more comprehensive information to families with whom they work.

Parent Education

Parent-education services involve the provision of information about the expected course of child development. Typical sequences of development, acceptable variations, anticipated difficulties in the presence of stressful events, and finding the right kind of help when the parent has questions or needs guidance can be subjects covered in parent-education programs. Such services can be provided in the context of a scheduled workshop or series of workshops or can involve use of a longer sequence of meetings (or even a formal academic course). A number of excellent commercial programs are available for implementing parent-education programs that the SLP may wish to review. Merely providing parents with information on child development and engaging them in problem solving has produced positive developmental outcomes in some cases.[3–6]

Generally speaking, few parents have had any formal coursework in child development; even fewer have had exposure to information about syndromes, diseases, anomalies, or other conditions their children may have. Information about expected variations in acquisition of communication skills, available treatment options, how to locate credentialed professionals, traditional and experimental or controversial approaches, legal entitlements and responsibilities, and how to locate parent-support groups or organizations that provide specific information about a given condition are examples of topics that could be covered in a more targeted parent-education program for families whose children are known to have (or to be at high risk for) developmental problems. Because the SLP has a broad understanding of available resources (e.g., printed materials, organizations, videotapes, and other educational materials), he or she may serve as a specialist in accessing the information parents need.

The costs of parent-education programs, including the time of professionals involved, an assigned share of operation costs of the facility, and materials and supplies, are sometimes contributed by an agency as part of their dedication to public awareness, information, and prevention. When that is not the case, families or a third-party payer (e.g., social-service agency, sponsoring organization that underwrites the service) may be charged an enrollment or tuition fee. A point to remember is that there *is* a cost to providing such programs.

Parent Training

Parent training is distinguishable from parent education in that it is directed toward parental acquisition of information and specific skills and strategies used in treatment regimes or management procedures delineated in the care plan for their child. For example, families of babies who are tube fed are trained by nursing professionals in appropriate procedures to complete the feedings. Such training includes such strategies as sterilization of the tube area and implements used in the feeding, prevention of common misapplications that result in stomach cramps, and management of bowel problems that can be associated with tube feedings. Children who are tube fed are often provided with nonnutritive sucking devices, so that normal motor coordination is established for the functions underlying speech develop in spite of the fact that food is not ingested orally. Parents of youngsters with tracheostomies, apnea monitors, supplementary oxygen, and other devices require training to anticipate emergencies and respond to them, to understand how their child's developmental patterns may be affected by the devices, and to implement compensatory strategies when appropriate.

The SLP with appropriate training and experience in specialized care strategies can be involved in providing parent training on feeding and swallowing; communication development in tracheostomized infants and toddlers; pre- and postsurgical counseling for families whose children have craniofacial disorders; and specific strategies to promote communication development for children with diagnosed diseases, conditions, and syndromes. Collaboration with other health professionals in parent-training efforts is often necessary when the nature of the child's problem is complex. Physical and occupational therapists can assist the SLP in advising parents about positioning of the child to optimize communicative efforts. Along with nurses and medical practitioners, they can help "read" infant signals that help adults interpret the baby's physical condition, state of alertness, and stress.

Of particular value to families of infants and young toddlers is training in specific techniques relating to (1) appropriate communicative stimulation and its timing, (2) techniques to calm a child (e.g., swaddling, positioning and handling to accommodate for hypersensitivity), and (3) optimizing attentiveness and interaction.

Direct billing for parent training is generally appropriate, but the manner in which billing procedures are handled can vary from one employment setting to the next. Some third-party payers require a physician order for such training; others may accept parent training as a standard protocol under certain conditions.

Direct Treatment and Management of Communicative Delays or Disorders

The SLP can be involved in direct treatment strategies necessitated by issues of the child's health and survival. Chapter 5 explores a number of such instances and elaborates on the SLP's role in the feeding and swallowing treatment plans for infants in the neonatal intensive care unit. Of particular importance in this discussion are issues concerning the scope of practice appropriate to specific professional disciplines, licensure stipulations (i.e., who is licensed by the state to do what), what constitutes best practices for the situation at hand, costs associated with specialized care, conservation of resources through staff collaboration, and competencies of individual staff members.

Many children with developmental delays or disorders can benefit from child-centered, family-focused management approaches that employ a range of activities and do not require a traditional clinical treatment regime. There are instances, however, when direct management or treatment of the child's communication problem is required. Examples of this situation include instances in which the child is in need of amplification, augmentative communication training, management of developing oral communication in the presence of a tracheostomy, or when implementation of compensatory strategies are necessary. Sometimes parents request direct treatment in the traditional model even when their children do not have such unusual problems. Families may prefer the privacy of the traditional clinical model.

After reviewing the array of treatments available, some parents conclude that a direct one-on-one therapeutic intervention protocol is optimal for their child. An example of this is the applied behavioral analysis approach (e.g., the

Lovaas method) for management of behaviors, including communicative behaviors associated with pervasive developmental delay and autism.

In most cases, application of direct treatment strategies does not necessarily eliminate access to additional forms of management. In many cases, direct treatment programs are administered in addition to or in conjunction with other management programs in which the child is enrolled.

Prevention

Prevention is an emerging and important role for the SLP. Families of children diagnosed with inherited conditions may wish to know the probability of bearing another child with the same disorder. In the case of primary prevention, when there is hesitancy about accepting a recommendation for genetic counseling, the SLP may assist other health care providers by listening to the concerns of the parents, providing appropriate information to them in layperson's terms, and allaying fears about the procedure of obtaining the necessary samples and subsequent medical counseling.

Placement of the discussion of prevention toward the end of the list of services the SLP provides or collaborates with other professionals in providing may seem strange. However, it is often the occurrence of one child's developmental problems that initiates parental interest in issues of preventing the recurrence of such problems in the future. The current explosion of knowledge about genetic problems, however, does not extend to other causes of communication disorders, and it is the SLP's knowledge of available resources in the professional literature that is sought by families. Language-learning disabilities, familial stuttering, and other communication difficulties experienced by very young children are examples of problems for which information on prevention can be sought.

Secondary prevention, in which the focus is on avoiding exacerbation of an existing problem, is certainly a strategy used by the SLP (e.g., in instances of early onset of dysfluencies). Strategies are routinely recommended to parents to reduce the probability that the dysfluencies will progress to true stuttering. Other examples include recommendations that toddlers who are only children be provided opportunities to play with age peers to increase their need or desire to communicate and that parents reduce the level of language used with their children who are experiencing delayed language development. The latter, of course, is intended to provide appropriate speech models the children find easier to emulate.

Tertiary prevention is the application of therapeutic strategies to eliminate or modify an existing disorder and has been discussed in Chapter 2 (see The Concept of Prevention).

Application of Part H/Part C Intervention Mandates

Throughout this section, *Part H/Part C* is used to refer to strategies the SLP and others employ in their implementation of early intervention as mandated by federal statute and companion legislation in participating states. Under the Part H/Part C system, services must be provided in accordance with the IFSP. Thus, the SLP, as a member of the early intervention team, can provide a wide range of the services in one or more designated settings.

Home-based services are considered optimal for early intervention, because young children and their families have daily routines in which developmental stimulation can be implemented without setting aside "special" times or excluding other members of the family. The ability of individual family members to participate directly in intervention activities is a natural function of family interaction. Communication development typically occurs during the child's experiences in the natural environment of the home and with familiar people in that environment. Thus, meal times, bath time, routines of dressing and grooming, and other day-to-day experiences can be the "vehicle" for communicative development.

Many children spend a significant amount of time in child care settings, either homes in which a few children are cared for while parents work or larger centers licensed to care for many children across a range of ages. Such settings are also considered to be "naturalistic settings" under the law. Hence, many SLPs provide direct services, indirect services, or both to children in these environments. It is important to keep in mind that most states require that directors of such centers possess credentials that reflect their knowledge of child development, but it is also true that the minimum requirements for child care workers employed in the centers are generally proof of having reached a minimum age (often 18 years), a health certificate verifying that the worker is free of communicable diseases, and basic understanding of universal precautions and the requirements for reporting child abuse and neglect. Strategies described above in the sections on parent education and parent training can be adapted by the SLP in working collaboratively with employees of child care agencies. Consultation services, demonstration of specific strategies, and assistance in devising efficient records relating to the child's communication development behaviors can be appropriate means of extending care through the child's daily activities and caregivers.

Some Head Start centers and school districts have established programs for infants and toddlers with special needs. If Part H/Part C services are offered through those entities, employers are required to adhere to hiring "qualified providers" as defined under the statutes. Early interventionists and teachers who work in those settings are likely to have had more exposure to formal educational programs relating to early childhood development and to be required to participate in ongoing professional development programs. It is wise to bear in mind, however, that personnel shortages often necessitate the hiring of uncertified individuals. (Unfortunately, in some states the proportion of uncertified to certified personnel approaches 50%.) SLPs working in those settings should be sensitive to the needs of employees who work with at-risk infants and toddlers and tailor their strategies to use staff strengths and be responsive to areas in which the need for information, education, and training are identified.

There are many dedicated, effective, and caring individuals who work in daycare settings and early-intervention programs throughout the country. Collaboration with staff members extends care through the efforts of staff members and in the daily activities of children enrolled in those settings.

Special Features and Requirements of Part H Early Intervention

Compliance with several requirements of Part H legislation should be noted by the SLP:

1. The IFSP must be reviewed and updated at least every 6 months and before that if conditions warrant or a parent requests the review or a change in its provisions.
2. When the child approaches the age of 3 years, transition planning is required. A change in the setting in which services are provided, personnel providing the services, and programs under which the child is (or is not) eligible to continue services must be identified. A plan of action to accomplish the transition from Part H services must be completed with the parent's participation.
3. Parents can choose at any time to participate or withdraw themselves, their child, or both from services recommended or actually undertaken. They can select those services they believe will help them optimize their child's development, even if the professional recommends another approach or priority.
4. Access by professionals to payment for services rendered is dictated by the state's Part H system. Some court cases have prohibited states from accessing the family's private insurance, if payments from those funds jeopardize the family's ability to maintain that coverage or burden the family in other ways with respect to their future access to that coverage.

National Effort to Make a Difference for Infants and Toddlers with Special Needs

Despite occasional difficulties in meeting timelines, navigating Part H/Part C rules and regulations, and keeping abreast of the ongoing process of legislative reauthorization with its attendant procedural modifications, Part H/Part C has established national recognition of the importance of early intervention for children with special needs. Through substantial funding to participating states, it provides the means by which families that would otherwise be unable to obtain services for their at-risk infants and toddlers can access such care. Through judicial rulings, the Part H/Part C rights of families of very young children with developmental delays and disabilities have been affirmed. No other country in the world can boast such a record on behalf of their youngest and most vulnerable citizens.

BEST PRACTICES UNDER ALL
SERVICE-DELIVERY MODELS

Regardless of the specific service-delivery model or the set of strategies used by the SLP, individualization of intervention plans and attempts to help the young child acquire the power of functional communication are common features of effective treatment, management, and intervention. To those ends, best practices call for employment of qualified, credentialed personnel; application of appropriate strategies and techniques; collaboration among agencies and personnel for the benefit of the child; involvement of the family in planning and implementing care; adherence to standards of care and ethical practices; and personal dedication to the goal of helping the child achieve optimal communicative function.

PRACTICAL PROBLEM-SOLVING APPROACHES
FOR INFANTS AND TODDLERS WITH
DELAYED OR IMPAIRED COMMUNICATION

"I understand all that, but what do I *do*?" When that question comes up, as it inevitably does with students, there is only one correct answer: Identify the needs and solve the problem of how they can be met most efficiently. It has been the author's experience that this is not the answer students hope to get. Experienced practitioners, however, know that it is the only way to get things done. They also know that the fund of knowledge from which to draw in designing what to do comes from accumulated experience over time, with each experience contributing another bit of critical information to one's personal database. To say that one "does by doing" is an oversimplification, because it is the *integration* of information and experiences that leads the practitioner to make decisions that are likely to produce an effective treatment, management, or intervention plan.

Personnel employed in health care settings may be required to use standardized, agency-approved plan formats. These can take the form of notes in the medical chart, discharge plans, or other documents maintained in accordance with agency accreditation bodies. Copies of such procedural requirements may be available for individual practitioners who wish to compare what is done in other settings with their own. Some practitioners are required by their employers to use computerized forms for generating intervention plans. Sometimes the motivation for adopting such formats is to optimize the professional's planning time; sometimes it is to have data sets that are readily available for record keeping and monitoring purposes; sometimes it is done on the basis of personal preference. How much plan individualization is truly achievable is beyond the scope of this discussion.

Crais and Roberts[7] and Wetherby[8] have devised exemplary and complementary, but quite different, problem-solving formats by which the SLP can be guided in making critical therapeutic decisions. Crais and Roberts' "decision tree" approach helps the practitioner formulate what is known about a given child's communicative skills and follow binary choices regarding "next steps" in planning how to deal with the problem or problems. The tree is arranged to address the needs of prelinguistic children, with subsequent sections focusing on the needs of children with increasingly sophisticated communication skill levels. It is easy to use and helpful in explaining procedural decisions to parents.

Wetherby's approach is based on the research that led to development of the Communication and Symbolic Behaviors Scale (CSBS).[9] After completing an assessment of the child's communicative abilities and needs, she recommended completing a profile that pinpoints strengths, weaknesses, and recommendations with reference to the child's communicative functions, communicative means (i.e., gestural, vocal, and verbal), reciprocity, social-affective signaling, and symbolic behavior. The method is adaptable to any means of assessing the child's communicative abilities, although the examiner may have to recast the resulting data into the definitional categories used with the CSBS. A statement of the differential diagnosis, if available, is also recorded.

Once that process is completed, the next step in Wetherby's approach is to prioritize intervention goals for children with emerging language. Goals are set for both the child and for the communication partner. A portion of a sample plan for an infant with limited skills, for example, may include (p. 11)[8]:

Goal for learner: Expand use of social-affective signals.

Goal for partner: Foster facilitative interaction style.

Strategies: Adult should follow child's lead by imitating child's behavior and attuning to child's display of affect. Use proximity in positioning and presentation of materials to enhance social referencing.

Use of this problem-solving approach to developing individualized plans allows the practitioner a great deal of latitude in providing clearly worded functional goals preserving considerable variety in the means by which the goals can be implemented. The goals can be selected jointly by the family and the SLP. Attaining the goal can include strategies that involve parent education regarding the expected types of responses the child may exhibit; parent training involving demonstration of specific techniques that could be used during different caregiving and play routines; and easy ways to document what was tried and the results, so that the professional can monitor progress from visit to visit.

Excerpts from a plan for a toddler with more advanced emerging communication may include the following (p. 11)[8]:

Goal for learner: Enhance symbolic level from presymbolic communication to referential language, from nonlinguistic comprehension strategies to linguistic comprehension, from exploratory actions on objects to functional object use and single and multiple action schemes toward self and others, and from exploratory actions to combinatorial actions to construct a simple product.

Goal for partner: Adjust language input to match and be slightly above child's language level and provide "scaffolding" to foster learning.

Strategies: Provide opportunities to engage child in appropriate use of objects and to model play at appropriate level for child during a variety of symbolic and constructive play experiences. Provide developmentally appropriate activities and use areas of relative strength to enhance areas of weakness (e.g., types of play, communicative functions); when play demands are more difficult for child, minimize communicative demands, but model and prompt developmentally appropriate behaviors.

Note that the format remains the same for developing the plan and that the plan is not cast in terms of traditionally worded behavioral objectives (e.g., given a situation in which a vocalized "request" is expected, the child will demonstrate the ability to spontaneously initiate inflected vocalization a minimum of 15 times in 20 consecutive opportunities). Wetherby's emphasis is on functional communicative skills rather than on task-specific criteria. This change in emphasis is in keeping with practices with which managed care providers (insurers) are familiar: functional goal attainment. By definition, *functional goals* relate to skills that can be applied across a variety of situations as opposed to discrete applications to designated situations. Readers who are interested in more information about functional treatment outcomes can obtain a packet of materials on the topic from the American Speech-Language-Hearing Association.[10]

FITTING SPECIFICS INTO THE TREATMENT AND INTERVENTION FRAMEWORK

Facilitating Communicative Development in Infancy

The focus of services during the early months is to promote the family's ability to (1) understand and encourage interactions between the infant and caregivers, (2) facilitate the child's physical development to support preverbal vocalization and other forms of communication, (3) provide opportunities for cognitive development, (4) support any special care that is necessitated by the child's condition, and (5) monitor and report changes in the child's physical and behavioral status. Ongoing assessment of the child's communicative development is also an important contribution of the SLP to these efforts. As practitioners work with families in their homes or center-based programs, with child care workers in daycare centers, and with other communicative partners of the child, it is imperative that cultural issues be considered. Customs, preferred languages, and attitudes about expected interactions among adults and children can be different from those that seem natural to an SLP with a different cultural background. Adaptations of the suggestions presented in Facilitating Interactions Between the Infant and Caregivers, below, may be required, although most are acceptable to families who are members of most cultures.

Facilitating Interactions Between the Infant and Caregivers

The SLP must have access to the child's caregivers to be able to provide information to those with whom the infant interacts. In some families, the only caregiver is the mother; in others, both parents are caregivers; in others, caregiving is provided by personnel at a child care center. Older siblings, members of the extended family, in-home sitters, or home-health professionals may also interact with the baby on a regular basis. With the help of the family, it can be determined who needs the information and how it can be provided to them most effectively.

The next step is to decide what information it is necessary to provide. This varies from situation to situation and is largely dependent on how much information the caregivers already have about infant development and physical, cognitive, social, and communicative expectations. Subjects selected for discussion can include the following:

- The baby's state-regulation abilities and the "rhythms" or cycles associated with daily activities involving the baby and family
- How to "read" the baby's signals (e.g., evidence of stress, readiness to interact)
- The importance of talking to the baby, especially if the infant's condition is predictive of limited ability to provide the same quality of response or reward to the adult's efforts to interact
- The concept of dyads (partnerships) in interactions and providing opportunities for turn taking by the baby
- Management of social routines, that is, creating brief opportunities for interaction during caregiving activities without creating overstimulation, fatigue, or aversive reactions
- The importance of sharing information about communication with other family members and caregivers

The underpinnings of receptive language development are obviously operative from the earliest exposure to interaction with caregivers. The SLP may wish to stress that infants with adequate hearing and cognitive ability can discern the difference between similar phonemes and intonation patterns used by caregivers. Informative videotape recordings or printed handouts can be used as part of the family training and education effort. Such materials can be developed for a particular set of circumstances, or commercially available products can be used.

Facilitating Physical Development to Promote Readiness for Communication

The transactional linkage between physical development and communicative development is not always evident to caregivers. It may, therefore, be necessary to provide information about the important relationship between a child's physical health and maturation and ongoing communicative development. Topics that the SLP may wish to cover in this connection include the following:

- Feeding as a pleasurable experience, especially with reference to oral-motor stimulation. For children who are tube-fed, nonnutritive sucking can be used to simulate this pleasurable experience.
- Handling and positioning the baby to enhance physical development. If the infant is physically handicapped, the information given to parents should be chosen in consultation with the infant's physician or physical or occupational therapist. Babies who are prenatally exposed to drugs need specific handling techniques to assist in behavioral organization. If the family was given instructions regarding physical handling at the time of hospital discharge, reconfirming their importance can be helpful.
- Respiratory considerations can also require special handling, positioning, or supportive technology. Consultation with other members of the child's multidisciplinary team may be required to address this issue appropriately. Babies with a combined history of bronchopulmonary dysplasia and intraventricular hemorrhage are at significant risk for development of communicative disorders.
- Care of the ears and information about the importance of seeking prompt care for ear infections is probably a topic that should be included in all early parent-education and parent-training plans because special-needs babies as a group have a significantly higher risk of developing frequent ear infections. Caregivers of infants with craniofacial anomalies should be especially alert for such problems, and they may require instruction on how to position the child during feedings to avoid leakage of fluids into the eustachian tubes. Propping bottles should be discouraged for all infants, not only because of potential ear infections but also because it deprives the infant of important tactile stimulation, mutual gaze with the adult during feedings, and early turn-taking interactions that promote communicative development.
- Visual impairment and adaptations for stimulation. Babies with known visual impairment often lack the richness of environmental stimulation available to other children during infancy. Compensation for the reduced visual stimulation should begin early. The infant can benefit from enhanced auditory and tactile stimulation. Care should be given in selecting objects for exploration on the basis of variations in size and texture. (Hint: Surface patterns can be raised by outlining them with nontoxic "puff paint" so that they can be felt.) Scent, weight, temperature, and auditory properties of materials can also be varied. The baby should be stimulated to use residual vision, even if it is severely limited. Sensory interactions between the infant and caregiver can include plac-

ing the baby's hand on the side of the partner's nose or on the lips or larynx as speech is produced, so that the baby can feel vibrations and movement associated with speech.

Facilitating Cognitive Development

Many caregivers are content to allow a quiet, compliant child to be left undisturbed. There may be little understanding of the importance of exposing the child to a range of experiences to promote cognitive development. Classic studies of children in orphanages in the United States during the 1930s and studies done in Romania in the late 1980s and early 1990s testify to the ravages that "benign neglect" have on infant development. It is particularly critical that infants at risk for mental retardation receive regular stimulation from other people. During caregiving routines and periods of purely social interaction, it is relatively easy to establish stimulating experiences that enhance cognitive development. The SLP may wish to provide information to caregivers about ways to provide the following:

- Appropriate tactile stimulation—through handling, positioning, touch, and pressure. This is especially important with children who have or are at risk for cerebral palsy and for those who have had prenatal drug exposure.
- Appropriate visual stimulation—by varying the baby's opportunities to view shapes, colors, light, shadows, and movement. It may be appropriate to provide information to caregivers about the importance of visual acuity to cognitive, social, and communicative development. Consultation with the physician or vision specialist is appropriate before providing any information of this nature if the infant is known to be visually impaired.
- Appropriate auditory stimulation—by providing opportunities for the child to hear a variety of sounds throughout the day and by avoiding exposure to excessively loud noises, including amplified music. Even from the earliest weeks, the infant is able to separate the human voice and many of its variations from other sounds in the environment. It is from consistent exposure to the sounds of speech that the child begins to build an awareness that strings of sounds are means of communication and to discern the fundamental phonemes of the language of the home. Early in life, emotional content is perceived by the child as it is conveyed by intonation and stress patterns used by the adult. In fact, intonational patterns emerge quite early in the child's own vocalization patterns. Surprisingly, the importance of giving the infant opportunities to hear the human voice is not universally known. Children who spend long hours away from the mother in child care settings can benefit from having the mother's tape-recorded voice available at times of stress or to soothe them to sleep. Family members or others charged with providing

care to an especially fussy baby or one who is difficult to console may also find that a tape recording of the mother reading a story, singing, talking on the phone, or uttering comforting phrases has a calming effect. The SLP may wish to consult the infant mental-health literature for specific information about the importance of the tone of voice used by caregivers who influence the child's development of a sense of emotional security.

- Appropriate motor stimulation—which is associated with cognitive development. Babies with atypical physical development benefit from information prepared by physical and occupational therapists with respect to motor stimulation. Some children profit from application of neurodevelopmental and sensory integration techniques. Collaboration with motor development specialists is productive.

- Opportunities to experience different environments—both indoors (different rooms of the house) and outdoors where sights; sounds; lights and shadows; and features of the sky, wind, and earth change with the time of day and season of the year is healthy. An exception to encouraging environmental variety, of course, applies when the child's health is at significant risk. If that exception does not apply, it is probable that confining children to a limited environment because of atypical physical features or the caregiver's anticipation of personal stress is unwarranted.

The sense of security that is so important in infancy and that allows the child to enjoy a variety of experiences from an early age derives, at least in part, from the baby's relationship with primary caregivers.[11-13] Sparks[11] discussed this in terms of "goodness of fit" between the baby and (initially) the mother. Zeanah and colleagues[12] referred to the phenomenon as *infant attachment*. The baby's sense of security is also related to development of a sense of the rhythms of the total environment, which some practitioners refer to as the child's *ecosystem*. Infants who exhibit significant and persistent difficulty in adjustment are likely to have difficulties with cognitive, social, and communication skill development. When such problems are noted by the SLP, collaboration with the child's physician or mental-health specialist is in order.

Severe difficulty in psychobehavioral adjustment is a characteristic of many children who were exposed prenatally to cocaine and other drugs. It is also characteristic of children with certain psychopathologies, such as autism. Sometimes medical or nutritional problems are implicated. For those reasons, persistent problems with adjustment should be investigated with the utmost care by appropriately selected specialists.

Supporting Special Care Necessitated by the Child's Condition

Children with a wide variety of handicapping conditions require special care, a portion of which is related directly to promoting communicative development. Obvious examples are children with cleft lip and palate, congenital hearing impairment, or "floppy" muscle tone; babies who exhibit hypersensitivity to sensory stimuli; infants who are excessively irritable or difficult to console; very low birth weight babies; and babies with diagnosed syndromes. It is essential that the SLP be sensitive to the fact that the family undergoes a tremendous amount of stress when they learn their child has special problems. Their receptivity to and desire for information pertinent to the baby's condition varies significantly within and across families. Even the *same* family member may relate to the professional on different levels at different times, depending on the stresses and concerns that affect the adult at a given moment and on that person's means of coping with them.

The SLP who is involved with the treatment and management of children with significant impairments may need to assist the family with incorporating communicative interventions with care prescribed by other members of the multidisciplinary team. Attempts to do this should always be accompanied by an appreciation for the family's priorities and their readiness to interact both on a personal level with the SLP and on a subjective and emotional level with the management plan per se.

Providing the family with information about available resources can be helpful (see Appendix C). Assisting them in understanding technical terms that other professionals may use and fail to explain can also be a way of assisting. Any family, but especially those dealing with the stresses of decision making for a child with extensive special needs, is only able to absorb so much information at one time. Being considerate by giving information that is a priority at the moment and reserving the rest for a later meeting helps families retain important data and reassures them that additional information will be made available when they indicate that they are ready for it.

Depending on the condition(s) the child possesses, the SLP may need to be prepared to provide information in the following areas:

- Respiration and respiratory functions for speech
- Special feeding considerations
- Positioning and handling the baby for optimal interactions
- Physical therapy and occupational therapy
- Presurgical and postsurgical care
- Communication considerations during recovery
- Overt physical and cognitive limitations
- Expectations for atypically developing children

Monitoring Changes in Physical and Behavioral Status

Because communicative development is so intimately interwoven with all facets of a child's development, it is essential that the other aspects of maturation be monitored and that the SLP have knowledge of what is happening with the whole child. To this end, the SLP may ask the family to engage in specific activities that provide a summary of pertinent information that can be incorporated into the management-planning process. Some information is available from formal reports of other professionals who see the child. However, the time lag between requests for reports and their receipt can slow down the process of efficient monitoring and interfere with planning efforts. For that reason, certain information can be monitored and recorded by the family using a checklist or other simple form to report observed changes in the following:

- Physical growth—by recording the baby's weight at specified intervals or at the time of regular health care visits
- Maturation—by recording attainment of specified milestones (e.g., sitting independently, responding to his or her name, crawling, pulling to stand, cruising)
- Behavioral characteristics—by recording new behaviors that are significant in communicative development as they emerge (e.g., cooing, babbling, emergence of first word)
- Plateaus or reversals in development—by recording, in anecdotal form, any apparent lack of progress that can signal a need for attention from the SLP or other members of the multidisciplinary professional team or a need to revise the intervention and treatment plan. The SLP should alert the parents to expected plateaus (e.g., reduction in vocalization during rapid acquisition of major physical milestones). Reversals in development can be of great significance and should be noted.

The system of collecting information should be simple and clearly specified. Parental preferences should be honored. The SLP or multidisciplinary team may wish to provide the materials for record keeping (e.g., charts, checklists, forms, notebook or journal). Some multidisciplinary teams have developed booklets that can be tucked into the mother's purse or diaper bag and be readily available for visits to the doctor's office, as well as being accessible to team members in their offices or on home visits.

The tasks requested of parents in connection with record keeping should be reasonable in terms of time requirements and simplicity (excessively detailed information requires time and effort to generate). New parents seldom have either extra time or abundant energy. When the child is at risk or has a diagnosed condition, the conditions may be doubly stressful and reduce the probability that record keeping will be done. The parents' reading level and familiarity with English are also considerations. Acknowledgment of their efforts should be provided by members of the professional team. The family needs to know that they are regarded as important participants in their child's program of care and that information they supply is valuable in planning and evaluating the effectiveness of that program.

Treatment, Management, and Intervention with Toddlers

At 12–14 months of age, children are classified as toddlers whether or not they are physically capable of walking. The designation presumes exposure to an array of life experiences and a certain degree of developmental maturation. Children with severe disabilities are less likely to have attained the milestones achieved by their typically developing peers in either physical or communication domains. Even in children who exhibit no overt disability, some fail to develop satisfactory receptive communication, expressive communication, or both. Most, however, have developed at least a meager understanding of the efforts made to communicate with them and have at least some form of expression, whether it be eye gaze to indicate a choice, pointing and grunting to make a request, gesturing, inflected vocalizations, or true efforts to use words. A determination of whether a child's expressive communication is merely delayed or is probably disordered is possible even before the second birthday (see Chapter 7). That determination assists in guiding the specific techniques applied in the treatment and management plan for an individual child.

Adult Instruction

Because parents and other adult caregivers are intimately involved in meeting the needs of atypically developing infants and toddlers, it is important that the SLP understand not only child development, assessment, and treatment protocols but also have a working knowledge of the principles of adult education. Effectiveness of any treatment or management plan to achieve communication goals for the child depends to a large extent on how effectively the SLP succeeds in collaborating with adults who interact regularly with the child. This involves both imparting needed information to them and assisting them with development of specific skills.

Adult instruction includes some or all of the following:

- Provision of written materials about the child's diagnosed condition, developmental expectations, and other pertinent matters
- Provision of information about the developmental stage at which their child presently functions
- Demonstration of specific techniques
- Discussion of the use of play and family routines as vehicles for communicative development
- Observation of the efforts of parents and caregivers in implementing recommended practices or techniques
- Coaching of parents and caregivers when adjustments are indicated and affirming and praising what they do that engages the child and results in communicative interaction

To minimize costs, groups can be formed for such instruction when appropriate. The Hanen program[14] for parent training is an example of a successful program designed for groups of parents. Other such programs are available for children with special needs and can be obtained through commercial vendors. Most programs of this nature need to be supplemented to address specific needs of a given child and family, but a great deal of well-developed material cast in excellent, well-researched formats is available.

Late Talkers

One of the most rewarding aspects of early communication intervention is seen with children who are late talkers. They are the children who have no other known problems but demonstrate delay in the onset and development of speech. They exhibit, at age 24 months, fewer than 50 words in their expressive vocabularies and have no two-word combinations. They may have had an ear infection once or twice, but they do not have histories of chronic otitis media. Their receptive language appears to be intact.

For such children, a short-term treatment program can be very effective. The program should include child assessment to ensure that the child meets criteria for group IV (risk 0) (see Table 7.2). The program should focus on parent instruction in turn-taking strategies, imitation and expansion of the child's utterances, pretending, and repetition strategies. Striking improvement in late-talking toddlers' communicative abilities usually occurs during or shortly after parent enrollment in such programs.[6] If the children do not have regular opportunities to interact with age peers, participation in a play group, mother's-day-out, or nursery-school program can be indicated. Direct therapy provided by professionals is generally not indicated for these children

Assistive Technology

For some children, even those who do not have hearing loss, a treatment of choice is early introduction of assistive communication. Early amplification for children who can benefit from it is certainly indicated (see Chapter 9). Toddlers diagnosed with impairments affecting gross motor development and those with oral motor apraxia may be candidates for assistive communication approaches. Depending on the characteristics of the impairments, choices range from early introduction of sign language, pairing adult speech with fingerspelling or using a total communication approach, introduction of electronic switches in operation of toys (later switch operation can be used with electronic communication devices), and the use of simple communication boards constructed to meet the needs of the child at a particular time (e.g., postsurgical hospitalization).

Children for whom assistive communication therapy is appropriate should experience a high degree of impact when they exert the effort to use the chosen approach. Their partners' responses to their expressions of intent should be prompt and appropriate. Attribution of presumed intent should be offered by the adult when it is apparent that the child is attempting to use the assistive method to communicate. When it is clear that the intent is to express a choice, make a request, offer an observation, convey feelings, affirm or negate, or offer information, it is important that communicative partners verbalize their understanding of the child's intent. This not only recognizes the attempt to convey a particular intent but also allows the child to affirm or deny the partner's interpretation of intent. Typically developing peers enjoy the rewards of affecting events in their lives; that power also enhances the communicative development of atypically developing children.

Use of assistive devices, of course, must be determined in light of the child's apparent cognitive abilities. Development of a sense of cause and effect (e.g., when the water is running, bath time is approaching; when a bottle or feeding equipment appears, a meal is on the way) can indicate a toddler's readiness for introduction to switches that cause toys to do something. To the extent possible, the assistive system should support later verbal communication if it is anticipated that the child will develop it at some point. It should enable the child to communicate with as many individuals as possible. It should be paired with the partner's use of speech so that associations can be established between verbal symbols (e.g., words, phrases) and the symbols used in the assistive method used.

Toddlers, even those who are physically challenged, learn best through play and the interactions of daily living. Thus, efforts to support development of communication should be focused on such activities and at a level on which the child is able to function. The reader may wish to refer to Appendix B and the suggestions developed by Norris and Hoffman[15] for children functioning below a developmental age of 1 year.

A Word about Toddlers with a History of Brain Injury in Infancy

Children who have a history of brain injury in early infancy appear to need more frequent exposures to language experiences in early childhood to attain normal levels of language ability.[16] Encouraging multiple exposures to such experiences can be viewed as a form of prevention or amelioration of future language problems for which the child is at risk. As time goes on, the need for such added exposure, combined with pressures to master specific material in the classroom under time constraints, can reveal previously unsuspected learning difficulties. Therefore, as these children enter school or center-based programs, continued monitoring is recommended and should be communicated to personnel in those settings.

Approaches When Assistive Technology Is Not Required

For purposes of the following discussion, it is assumed that the child for whom a program is being planned has demonstrated some cognitive ability, has attending behaviors that allow the child to focus on tasks that interest him or her, and has shown some frustration with his or her inability to communicate so that others can understand his or her intent. Such a child may be language delayed or language disordered. Ongoing assessments concurrent with treatment and intervention discriminate between the alternative conclusions as the plan is implemented.

Direct Management
In planning ways to assist a child who has communicative difficulties, the SLP must address the following:

- The child must have experiences to which the symbols of communication can be applied.
- Communicative treatment or intervention should be interwoven with activities of daily living and not be a set of activities set aside for only specific blocks of time.
- Parents and caregivers should be directly involved in ongoing language-stimulation activities with the child.
- The plan of treatment or intervention must include strategies for adult education on how to provide effective interactions that are geared to the child's developmental level.
- Depending on the child's developmental level, language intervention can be directed at some or many of the following items:

    Labeling or naming objects, actions, feelings

    Attributing *meaning* to the child's actions

    Self-talk to describe one's own actions as they occur

    Parallel talk to describe the child's actions as they occur

    Providing *communicative temptations* that increase the probability that the child will attempt to communicate (see Appendix B for Wetherby's[8] list of communicative temptations).

    Making sure the child has a *need* to talk. Avoid the temptation to supply responses for the child when others ask questions or make comments directed to him or her.

    Positioning the child to optimize communicative events. Provide stable seating that minimizes the child's need to focus energies on balance. Place objects within reach if joint attention is desired. Place them just out of reach and stay near the child to optimize the probability of the child's requesting them.

    Withholding a desired object until the child attempts to communicate a desire for it. Avoid requiring the child to produce a target word perfectly. Reward attempts to verbalize.

    Assuring the power of communication. Be sure something *happens* when the child communicates; the attempt should have an effect.

    Engaging in vocal play. Just producing sounds for the fun of it is interesting to toddlers; varying intonation and stress patterns as the "game" proceeds highlights use of suprasegmental linguistic features. Be sure to imitate the child's vocalizations, taking turns in the vocal play as it progresses. Maintain the child's interest at an appropriate developmental level.

    Stimulating approximations of syllabic content. Avoid early attention to articulatory accuracy and focus on syllable configurations. This activity also enhances awareness of morphemes that are markers for number, tense, ongoing action, and possession. It also builds awareness of monosyllabic and polysyllabic elements.

    Producing meaningful nonspeech sounds such as motor noises, animal noises, and other environmental noises. These are often easier,

and sometimes less stressful, vocalizations that are early representations of the objects or actions with which the child is familiar.
Such intentional vocalizations can also be modified to include
emphasis, to imply a question, or to contrast qualities of loud or
soft speech.

Using mutual experiences in play that stimulate communicative interaction, such as splashing at bath time and banging on inverted plastic
containers to emulate the bang of a drumbeat or to establish rhythm
patterns that can be mirrored in vocalizations or verbalizations. This
is sometimes helpful in establishing syllabic configurations.

Simplifying adult language so that its flow is easier for the child to
follow (e.g., reduce sentence structure to basic elements, such as
"Bobby stand up," "Mary eat cookie," or "Mama go to store")

Accompanying verbalization with gestures or signs. This is helpful
even for some children who are not hearing impaired and especially for those who may have oral apraxia, pervasive developmental disorder (PDD), or central auditory processing difficulties.

Pairing speech with music or rhythm by singing, clapping, and speaking to phrase cadence

Enlisting the assistance of all members of the family to interact with
the child using the strategies that have been selected to interweave
communicative stimulation throughout the day's activities

Providing affective vocal models that show the child in play activities
how to express frustration and anger, as well as pleasure. A fact
that is poorly understood is that children who do not have symbolic means to express their emotions essentially have two choices:
withdraw or act out. Acting out often results in the interpretation
that the child has a behavior problem rather than a communication problem.

Using or adapting techniques designed for children with hearing
impairment when appropriate. Many activities recommended for
hearing-impaired children include appropriate techniques for language delayed and impaired children. Multisensory stimulation
and use of household objects and activities (e.g., responding to the
ring of a phone or doorbell, listening for the whistle of the tea ket-
tle) to focus joint attention are examples.

Following the child's lead and demonstrated interests. By their nature,
toddlers are explorers and do not have lengthy attention spans. As
their attention is attracted by objects and activities, be responsive
to the naturally occurring shifts and move along with them to
implement appropriate communicative activities.

Ongoing Assessment as Treatment or Intervention Planning

Ongoing assessment of the child's overall development and communicative
skills should guide the SLP and family in selecting appropriate goals for a given

time frame. Whether the child's needs dictate use of assistive communication; development of basic concepts; development of oral-motor or other physical competencies necessary to communicative skills; collaboration with other professionals in management of persistent sucking, swallowing, and feeding problems; development of auditory awareness and joint attention; or other targets, the SLP can help parents capitalize on the rich opportunities for stimulation that exist in daily activities.

SUMMARY

Many strategies can be used to assist children in acquiring communication skills, but the SLP who selects wisely from the approaches listed in this chapter can help the family and caregivers get started on a constructive program. The SLP needs to monitor progress, confer frequently with the family, evaluate circumstances as they change, and adjust the prescribed program as needed.

For most children, progress will occur if the following are true:

1. There are a sufficient number of attempts at communication; if there are not, increasing the attempts becomes a goal.
2. The child has a sense of security from knowing his or her attempts will be accepted and responded to by those with whom communication is attempted.
3. Communication is a part of most daily activities and is not an effort restricted to "therapy" or "speech" time.
4. The effort to communicate has results and a perceived effect.

It is impossible to guarantee that children entrusted to the care of an SLP will achieve optimal communicative functions and succeed thereby in being physically, mentally, and emotionally healthy. However, our pledge to these children and their families is to work with them and with our professional colleagues to make possible that which is within our ability to achieve.

REFERENCES

1. Brazelton TB. Assessment in Early Infancy as an Intervention. In D Gilderman, D Taylor-Hershel, S Prestridge, J Anderson (eds), The Health Care/Education Relationship. Chapel Hill, NC: Technical Assistance and Development System, 1981;3.
2. Coleman PP, Buysse V, Scalise-Smith DL, Schulte AC. Consultation: applications to early intervention. Infants Young Child 1991;4:41.
3. Banigan RL. Memorandum to the author, 1991.
4. Barrera M, Rosebaum P. The transactional model of early home intervention. Infant Ment Health J 1986;7:112.
5. Moxley-Haegert L, Serbin LA. Developmental education for parents of delayed infants: effects on parental motivation and children's development. Child Dev 1983;54:1324.
6. Schober-Peterson D, Cohen M. Facilitating Parent-Child Interactions. Paper presented at the ASHA Conference, Atlanta, November 1991.

7. Crais E, Roberts J. Decision making in assessment and early intervention. Language Speech Hear Serv Schools 1991;22:25.
8. Wetherby A. Infants and Toddlers with Special Needs. Syllabus accompanying presentation at the Alton Ochsner Clinic Continuing Medical Education Program, New Orleans, May 1996.
9. Wetherby AM, Prizant BM. Communication and Symbolic Behavior Scale (CSBS)–Normed Edition. Chicago: Applied Symbolix, 1993.
10. American Speech-Language-Hearing Association. Packet of Reports on Treatment Outcomes. Rockville, MD: American Speech-Language-Hearing Association, 1997. (Available from ASHA, 10801 Rockville Pike, Rockville, MD 20852.)
11. Sparks S. Assessment and intervention with at-risk infants and toddlers: guidelines for the speech-language pathologist. Top Lang Disord 1989;10:43.
12. Zeanah CH Jr, Mammen OK, Lieberman AF. Disorders of Attachment. In CH Zeanah Jr. (ed), Handbook of Infant Mental Health. New York: Guilford Press, 1993;332.
13. Letourneau N. Fostering resiliency in infants and young children through parent-infant interaction. Infants Young Child 1997;9:36.
14. Maolson, Ayala. It Takes Two to Talk (3rd ed). Toronto: Hanen Center Publications, 1992.
15. Norris JA, Hoffman PR. Comparison of adult-initiated vs. child-initiated interaction styles with handicapped prelanguage children. Lang Speech Hear Serv Schools 1990;21:28.
16. Keefe KA, Feldman HM, Holland AL. Lexical learning and language abilities in preschoolers with perinatal brain damage. J Speech Hear Disord 1989;54:395.

9

Habilitation and Communication Development in Hearing-Impaired Infants and Toddlers

Thomas G. Rigo

Hearing loss has a multidimensional effect on the communicative and social-emotional development of infants and toddlers. A hearing deficit early in life impairs the normal acquisition of speech and language. The communication problem can, in turn, cause learning and social difficulties, reduce academic performance, and limit vocational opportunities. The successful remediation of these potential deficits requires the collaborative efforts of speech-language pathologists (SLPs), audiologists, physicians, social workers, psychologists, educators of the deaf, and family members. This chapter discusses the effects of early hearing loss on communication ability and the procedures used to facilitate the development of speech and language. It focuses on those topics that relate directly to the typical functions of the speech-language pathologist and audiologist within the interdisciplinary framework.

EFFECT OF HEARING LOSS ON ORAL COMMUNICATION ABILITY

Sensory Perception

Speech sounds are composed of a combination of subphonemic features that give each sound its individual perceptual identity. Hearing loss disrupts the perception of speech by distorting or limiting the auditory reception of these features.

When a hearing loss occurs after language has developed (postlingual onset), a listener often is able to compensate for a loss of sensory input by predicting the likely components of a message. Once an elemental amount of sensory information is received, an understanding of the rules of language and the use of contextual and situational cues allow the listener to make predictions about the likely structure and content of the message. The acoustic pattern need not be processed in detail; its analysis proceeds only so far as is necessary to confirm the accuracy of the anticipated linguistic patterns.

When a hearing deficit occurs before language is acquired (prelingual onset), the loss of sensory information has a more disruptive effect. A young

179

child, unable to predict how a message evolves, must analyze sensory input in more detail to acquire and comprehend oral language. If this input is degraded substantially by hearing loss, the acquisition of language auditorily may not be possible. As such, the handicap associated with a hearing loss depends not only on its severity but also its time of onset.

Auditory Reception

Vowels Vowels are intense phonemes and account for much of the energy in the long-term spectrum of speech. Their identification requires the reception of the first and second vowel formants (F1 and F2, respectively). F1 frequency location is related inversely to the degree of articulatory constriction. It ranges from 250 Hz for high vowels to 850 Hz for low vowels. F2 frequency location is related to the front-back place of production. It ranges from 850 Hz for back vowels to 2,800 Hz for front vowels.[1] As a general rule, the amplitudes of vowel formants decrease as their frequency locations increase.

Hearing loss most often affects the reception of F2. F1 is more likely to remain audible, because it is higher in intensity and lower in frequency. Both formants should remain audible to children with mild-to-moderate hearing impairments. Severe hearing loss above 1,000 Hz limits the reception of F2. Because F2 for front vowels is lower in intensity and higher in frequency, they are more vulnerable to distortion than are back vowels. Severe-to-profound hearing loss across all frequencies impairs the reception of both F1 and F2 formants.

Consonants The perception of consonants requires the reception of acoustic cues associated with voicing, manner of production, and place of production. The primary voicing cue is the presence or absence of fundamental frequency, located in the 100- to 250-Hz frequency range.[1] Secondary features, such as voice onset time and phoneme duration, extend the frequency range of voicing cues to the 2,000 Hz region. Fundamental frequency is an intense cue and remains audible to all but severe-to-profound hearing-impaired listeners.

Each class of consonants (i.e., semivowels, nasals, fricatives, stops) contains an acoustic cue associated with its manner of production. Semivowels are distinguished by a formant-like energy pattern in the 300- to 400-Hz frequency region. Nasals are characterized by the presence of a band of harmonic energy located at 200–300 Hz (nasal murmur). Both fricatives and stops are composed of wide-band, aperiodic acoustic energy that is predominant at frequencies above 1,000 Hz. The difference between these two classes of sounds is related to their temporal characteristics. Fricatives are associated with a continuous, steady-state noise pattern. Stops are characterized by a transient burst of noise.[2] The acoustic cues for semivowels and nasals are intense, harmonic, and low in frequency. They remain audible until hearing loss reaches a severe-to-profound level. In contrast, the acoustic cues for fricatives and stops are less intense and aperiodic. Manner confusions between these classes of sounds are more common and occur with lesser degrees of impairment.

Voicing and manner cues alone do not provide a listener with enough acoustic information to identify individual phonemes. For example, the reception of nasal murmur allows the recognition of a sound as a nasal but does not provide sufficient information to determine which nasal phoneme was spoken. The reception of acoustic cues associated with place of production is necessary to distinguish phonemes that share the same manner of production. These cues generally are located at frequencies above 1,000 Hz and are, as a group, the least intense of the subphonemic features of speech.[2] The loss or distortion of place of production information is the most common speech-reception deficit experienced by hearing-impaired listeners. Difficulties occur with any degree of hearing loss and typically result in the perceptual confusion of phonemes within a class of sounds.

The reception of the acoustic cues associated with a phoneme does not insure its accurate identification. Phoneme recognition also requires a listener to distinguish the small acoustic variations that occur among different speech sounds. Sensorineural hearing loss causes not only a loss of audibility but also a reduction of frequency, intensity, and temporal discrimination ability. For this reason, phonemes that are audible but similar acoustically may not be distinguishable to a hearing-impaired child. Discrimination ability cannot be predicted solely on the basis of threshold information. It can be determined, however, by more structured assessment procedures, such as analysis of acoustic confusions, minimal-pairs testing, and age-appropriate measures of speech discrimination.

Visual Reception

Speechreading (or lipreading) enables a person to obtain linguistic information by watching the articulatory movements of a speaker's lips, tongue, and jaw. It can improve the comprehension of speech by providing sensory cues that are unavailable auditorily because of hearing loss or environmental degradation of the acoustic signal. The amount of linguistic information that can be obtained by speechreading is limited because speech is not transmitted visually as efficiently as it is auditorily. Sensory cues are restricted by (1) the poor visibility of many speech sounds, (2) the occurrence of sounds that look alike (i.e., homophones), (3) the rate of speech, (4) articulatory differences among speakers, (5) the effect of coarticulation on the visibility and stability of articulatory movements, and (6) environmental conditions (e.g., lighting, viewing angle, distance from the speaker).[3] Because sensory input is limited, the visual perception of oral language is highly dependent on the speechreader's language competence and inductive ability; that is, a speechreader must be capable of arriving at perceptual and conceptual closures when a substantial part of the sensory code is either missing or ambiguous.

The primary sensory cue that is available visually is place of production. Place information is retrieved by observing the motor patterns associated with the production of phonemes. These patterns can be organized into contrasting

Table 9.1   Visible Speechreading Movements under Ideal Viewing Conditions

Movement Pattern	Associated Phonemes
Vowels and diphthongs	
Lips puckered*	/u, ʊ, o͞o, ɝ/
Lips back*	/i, ɪ, e͞ɪ, ʌ/
Lips rounded*	/ɔ/
Lips relaxed to lips puckered*	/a͞ʊ/
Lips relaxed	/ɛ, æ, ɑ/
Lips rounded to lips back	/o͞ɪ/
Lips relaxed to lips back	/a͞ɪ/
Consonants	
Lip to teeth*	/f, v/
Lips puckered*	/w, hw, r/
Lips together*	/p, b, m/
Tongue between teeth*	/θ, ð/
Lips forward*	/ʃ, ʒ, ʧ, ʤ/
Teeth together	/s, z/
Lips back	/j/
Tongue up or down	/t, d, n, l/
Tongue back	/k, g, ŋ/

*Denotes that the movement pattern is highly visible.

groups called *visemes* and are shown in Table 9.1.[3] The viseme groups are arranged separately for vowels and consonants in their order of visibility. Those marked with an asterisk are highly visible and can be identified accurately by most speechreaders. The other visemes listed are not as easily perceived and may not be distinguishable under less than ideal viewing conditions.

Individual phonemes, with the possible exception of the /ɔ/ and /j/, cannot be identified solely by their visual motor pattern, because many sounds share the same place of articulation. For example, /p/, /b/, and /m/ cannot be distinguished on the basis of visual information only; additional information about their voicing and manner characteristics is needed to discriminate one from the others.

For many hearing-impaired children, the comprehension of speech is not possible under auditory-only or visual-only conditions. Auditory cues are missing or distorted because of the hearing deficit, and visual cues are incomplete because of the inherent limitations of speechreading. However, when speech is processed under an auditory-visual (bimodal) condition, the nonoverlapping cues provided by each modality can be combined to improve message comprehension.

Oral-Language Characteristics

Most children with congenital or prelingual hearing loss exhibit delays or deficiencies in the acquisition of oral language. Problems can occur in all areas of language, including morphology, syntax, semantics, and pragmatics.

The oral-language deficits of hearing-impaired children are related primarily to the severity of hearing loss, although skills vary among children with similar audiograms. Other factors of influence include the time of onset of the hearing loss, discrimination skills, the timing and benefit of amplification, and the ability to tolerate and use incomplete sensory data.[4]

The language problems of hard-of-hearing children increase with the degree of hearing loss but generally do not approach the deficits that typically occur with profound impairment. Language-acquisition patterns are similar for normal-hearing children and those with mild hearing loss, and for children with moderate hearing loss and severe hearing loss.[5] The language difficulties of hard-of-hearing children can, in most cases, be remediated successfully if intervention is provided early and with strong family support. For many deaf children, however, the lack of sufficient sensory input prevents the acquisition of language auditorily.

The language deficits of hard-of-hearing children also differ qualitatively from those demonstrated by deaf children. Hard-of-hearing children usually exhibit a language delay rather than a language disorder. That is, they acquire language in a normal developmental sequence but at a slower rate than their normal-hearing peers. They may also demonstrate premature plateaus of development, particularly in the morphosyntactic area. In deaf children, deviant language forms can accompany severe language delay. Their knowledge of words and meanings may be irregular and related more to teaching curricula than to natural language experience. Their productions may be characterized by agrammatical and nonsentence forms, such as omissions of major sentence constituents, absent or incorrect morphologic markers, and asequential word orders.[2,6] The common oral language deficits of hearing-impaired children are listed in Table 9.2.

Speech Characteristics

Severe-to-Profound Hearing Loss

The vocalizations of deaf and normal-hearing children cannot be differentiated until shortly after the onset of babbling. Deaf children babble, but their vocalizations differ from those of normal-hearing children in both quantity and quality. Hearing infants typically exhibit an increase in speech-like sounds and a decrease in nonspeech sounds with age, but both types of vocalizations decline in deaf children shortly after babbling begins. Deaf babies evidence a smaller variety of consonant sounds and produce fewer multisyllabic utterances than hearing babies. They tend to produce a high proportion of vocalizations containing glides and glottal stops.[7,8]

The vocalizations of deaf children beyond the babbling stage depend on the quality of their auditory experience. The early preverbal behaviors of the deaf generally consist of auditory and vocal elements, gestural elements, and observation of the speaker. With early and proficient use of amplification, a primarily auditory and vocal style can develop. However, when hearing aids are delayed or

Table 9.2 Common Oral-Language Characteristics of Hearing-Impaired Children

Vocabulary and word-class usage
  Reduced vocabulary
  Restricted knowledge of word classes, including the following:
    Overuse of nouns and verbs
    Omission or restricted use of function words

Semantics
  Restricted use of semantic operations
  Restricted use of abstract language forms
  Difficulty with words with multiple meanings

Syntax
  Omission or restricted use of bound morphemes
  Restricted knowledge of verb forms
  Overuse of subject-verb-object sentence structures
  Reduced sentence length
  Restricted knowledge and use of complex sentence forms
  Reduced syntactic quality (word omissions, inversions, substitutions, and additions)
  Agrammatical sentence forms

Pragmatics
  Passive communication style (reduced initiation of verbal interaction)
  Difficulty sustaining and repairing conversations
  Provision of ambiguous or uninformative responses

provide little benefit, auditory and vocal behaviors decrease and visual and gestural behaviors predominate.[9]

The speech of deaf children is characterized by severe and multiple deficits that involve both segmental and suprasegmental aspects. As a group, their speech intelligibility is poor, although it varies widely among individuals. Most studies have found the intelligibility of deaf speakers to be 20–40%.[6] Deviant speech characteristics are due mainly to the loss of auditory feedback but also can be caused by poor respiratory control and excessive laryngeal and articulatory tension. The common characteristics of the speech of the deaf are listed in Table 9.3.

Mild-to-Moderate Hearing Loss

Although any degree of hearing loss can cause errors of speech production, the speech of hard-of-hearing children resembles the productions of normal-hearing children more closely than that of the profoundly impaired. Most hard-of-hearing children produce intelligible speech. Their voice quality, suprasegmental production, and vowel articulation is comparable to normal-hearing children. The majority of speech errors involves the articulation of consonants and consonant blends. Sounds of low intensity, high frequency, or short duration are most commonly affected. Errors of substitution and distortion predominate, although other types of errors occur frequently and include omission

Table 9.3 Common Speech Characteristics of Deaf Children

Suprasegmental
    Pitch and intensity characteristics
        Inappropriate vocal pitch (usually higher than normal)
        Pitch breaks
        Phonetically linked pitch breaks (usually on high vowels)
        Monotone voice
        Inappropriate vocal intensity (too loud or too soft)
        Inability to vary vocal intensity across speaking situations
        Faulty stress pattern (may stress all vowel nuclei)
    Temporal characteristics
        Slow speaking rate
        Abnormal pause behavior (both between and within phrase)
        Increased duration of speech sounds and segments
    Voice quality
        Harshness, breathiness, and hypo- or hypernasality may occur alone or in
          combination

Segmental
    Vowels and diphthongs
        Substitution (most often involving tense/lax or near-neighbor vowels)
        Neutralization
        Reduction of diphthongs; diphthongization of vowels
        Nasalization
    Consonants
        Omissions
            Word position (most often on word-final consonants)
            Place of production (most often on back consonants)
        Manner substitutions
            Nasal/oral
            Voice/voiceless
            Stop for fricative (due to articulatory overconstriction)
        Place substitutions (related to visibility factors)
        Distortions
        Poor coarticulatory skills
        Omission of consonant blends

Other characteristics
    Poor respiratory control
    Glottalization and intrusive voicing
    Exaggerated lip and jaw movement

of final consonants; decreased production of voiced fricatives; and limited use of voiced, back, lingual consonants.[5,6,10]

AURAL HABILITATION

The primary goal of aural habilitation is to maximize the receptive and expressive communication abilities of hearing-impaired children. Remediation activities can include parent counseling and education (see Chapter 4), the fitting of hearing aids or other sensory devices, sensory training (auditory and visual), the development of language in oral or manual form, and the development of speech.[11]

Hearing Aids

Hearing aid selection and fitting should begin immediately after a child's hearing loss is identified and medical clearance for hearing aid use is obtained. It is an ongoing process that requires close observation of aided behaviors, parental support and involvement, and collaboration among professionals involved in the child's management. Several clinical decisions are made by the dispensing audiologist during the hearing aid selection process, including (1) the type of hearing aid and earmold to be worn, (2) whether binaural or monaural amplification should be used, and (3) the ideal electroacoustic characteristics of the device(s). It is probable that fitting adjustments will be necessary, as the child's reaction to and performance with the instruments are monitored during the early period of hearing aid use.

Hearing Aid Orientation

Once amplification has been obtained, it should be introduced in a gradual fashion. Most children accept hearing aids quickly, but some may require a longer period of adjustment. Downs[12] recommended the use of a 6- to 8-week orientation program for young hearing aid users. Others have argued that such schedules draw attention to the hearing aid and lengthen the adjustment process.[13] Rather than adhering to rigid timetables or ignoring them completely, it is best to view orientation recommendations as guidelines that can be shaped to suit a child's particular reaction to hearing aid use.

The factors that should be considered during the adjustment process include (1) the period of time that the hearing aid is worn, (2) the gain-control setting, and (3) the listening situation. Initially, hearing aids should be worn for short periods (e.g., 10–20 minutes) several times a day with the gain control at its minimal setting. The time of use should be increased in small steps until the hearing aid can be worn successfully throughout the entire day. The gain control can be increased gradually during the early stages of the adjustment period until its target setting is reached. At first, the hearing aid should be worn in pleasant, reinforcing listening environments that contain minimal levels of ambient noise. Aided listening situations can then be expanded progressively from controlled acoustic environments to those that include a more natural and complex array of auditory stimuli.

Parents should be provided with a written orientation plan that includes time guidelines and practical examples of appropriate listening situations.

Use and Care of Hearing Aids

A hearing aid can be an intimidating device, and its use can seem awkward at first. Because of this, a significant amount of training, encouragement, and technical support from the dispensing audiologist and other clinicians is necessary during the early period of intervention to insure that the hearing aid is being used and maintained properly. Every caregiver in regular contact with a young hearing aid user should be taught the following:

1. The parts of a hearing aid (e.g., microphone, on-off switch, volume control, battery compartment, earmold, and tubing)
2. The correct insertion of the battery; how long it lasts; how to check its voltage; precautions for its safe use
3. The correct insertion of the earmold and how to keep it clean
4. The proper position of the volume control
5. The causes of acoustic feedback and what to do if it occurs
6. What can damage a hearing aid (e.g., impacts, high temperatures, moisture, excessive dirt or dust, hair spray)

The condition and performance of a hearing aid should be monitored on a daily basis. A routine check also should be conducted by clinicians before each therapy session. This is particularly important in light of the consistent (and disappointing) findings of a number of investigations concerning the condition of hearing aids worn by school-age children. These studies, conducted over a 30-year period, found that 27–92% of children's hearing aids are malfunctioning at any given time.[14]

Some equipment is needed to carry out a hearing aid check, including a battery tester, a hearing aid stethoscope or earmold, a brush and wire loop to remove cerumen from the earmold, and a hand syringe to clean the tubing of the earmold. A complete hearing aid check consists of the following:

- A visual inspection of the hearing aid, tubing, and earmold
  Check hearing aid switches.
  Check tubing for stiffness, holes, or cracks.
  Check earmold for cerumen and moisture.
- A battery check
  Check battery voltage.
  Check battery contacts for corrosion.
  Check that battery door is closed securely.
- A listening check
  Check the quality of amplified sound.
  Check for excessive noise, intermittent signals, and acoustic feedback while tapping the casing of the hearing aid and rotating the volume control.
  Check for a smooth increase in gain as the volume control is rotated.

Parents can solve many of the problems that inevitably occur by learning simple troubleshooting techniques. Common problems include the use of batteries that are dead, weak, or inserted improperly in the battery compartment; switches turned to incorrect settings; and earmolds that are too small, inserted incorrectly, or blocked by cerumen or moisture. Most problems can be solved without visits to the dispenser's office by providing parents with troubleshooting charts and procedures.

Alternative Sensory Devices

Cochlear Implants

In most sensorineural hearing losses, it is the hair cells of the inner ear that are nonfunctioning rather than the fibers of the auditory nerve. The benefit provided by hearing aids can be insignificant for many profoundly hearing-impaired patients because of the extent of hair-cell damage. A cochlear implant is designed to bypass the nonfunctioning hair cells by applying electrical stimulation directly to the fibers of the auditory nerve. The system consists of an external microphone, a speech-processing unit, a transmitting wire or coil, and a surgically implanted receiver-stimulator and electrode array.

To be considered for implantation, a child must be profoundly hearing impaired and obtain no significant benefit from hearing aids (i.e., the inability to use aided hearing for speech perception). The child must be at least 2 years of age before implantation, primarily to permit time for diagnosis, evaluation, and determination of hearing aid benefit. Additional nonauditory criteria can include normal intelligence, the absence of additional handicaps that can affect the success of the implant, and evidence of family support.[15] The anatomical factors that influence selection and postsurgical success include the patency of the cochlea and degree of neural survival.[16]

Speech-perception abilities vary greatly among children with cochlear implants and can range from limited sound detection to open set word recognition. The success of an implant is related most closely to (1) the age at which deafness occurred, (2) the duration of deafness before implantation, (3) the neural survival in the cochlea, (4) the coding strategy used by the speech processor, (5) the child's rehabilitation, and (6) the level of parental and educational support.[16,17] Generally, the largest improvements have been observed in adults and children with postlingual hearing loss. Although most children with congenital or prelingual hearing impairments benefit from cochlear implants, they are slower to acquire auditory skills and can require 1–2 years of implant use before demonstrating improvements in speech perception.[18] Performance improvements have been measured for a range of behaviors, including sound detection, pattern recognition, preverbal communication, closed- and open-set speech recognition, speechreading, and speech production.[19,20]

Vibrotactile Sensory Aids

Vibrotactile aids transduce auditory signals into vibratory patterns on the skin. They are a noninvasive alternative for deaf children who derive negligible benefit from conventional amplification. Both single-channel and multichannel devices are in use. Single-channel aids provide primarily suprasegmental information and segmental voicing cues. Multichannel systems (or vocoders) provide these same low-frequency cues and can also transmit high-frequency components of speech, including frication and other manner of production cues.[21,22]

Although vibrotactile devices have been shown to improve the speechreading abilities, early vocal behaviors, phonetic repertoires, and syllabic productions of young deaf children,[23,24] they require teaching and learning strategies that are different from those used with auditory devices like hearing aids and cochlear implants. Often, children can only receive training and follow-up services in specialized centers that are limited in number and removed from school settings.[21] These difficulties have prevented the extensive use of vibrotactile instruments in the deaf population.

Language Development

Communication Methodologies

A variety of communication methodologies are being used to facilitate the language development of hearing-impaired children. The major approaches are outlined in Table 9.4. Each method has its proponents and detractors, but no single method has proven to be best for all children. As Davis and Hardick[2] explained, "the major decision for infants is whether or not the child should be exposed to some form of manual communication . . . in addition to spoken language" (p. 158).

In the 1970s, total communication (TC) replaced oralism as the most common communication methodology used in educational programs for the hearing impaired. Debate continues, however, between oral and TC practitioners about the use of manual communication and its effect on the development of oral language. Oral proponents argue that the simultaneous use of speech and signs inhibits the development of speech perception and production skills. TC proponents maintain that the early establishment of language, regardless of teaching modality, serves to facilitate the development of oral communication. Empirical investigations have failed to clarify these issues. Some studies have measured superior oral-language abilities in children from oral programs,[25] whereas others have suggested that the use of a simultaneous communication technique is not a detriment to the development of oral-language skills.[26]

There is a general consensus that a unisensory or multisensory oral English method is most appropriate for hard-of-hearing children. For deaf children, however, the selection of the ideal educational approach is not as clear cut. The oral-language potential of deaf children depends not only on the amount of residual hearing but also on the age of onset, the age of identification and initiation of intervention, and the benefit provided by sensory devices. Other nonauditory factors can be of significant influence, including the child's cognitive ability, the existence of other handicapping conditions, the level of family support, and the types and quality of programs that are available in the child's community.[2]

Table 9.4 Communication Methodologies for Hearing-Impaired Children

Methodology	Description
Oral English	Reception and expression of language via speech Auditory reception can be supplemented by speechreading, other visual cues, or both.
Unisensory method (also known as *acoustic, auditory,* or *acoupedic*)	Uses auditory input only for speech perception Lipreading is discouraged until the child has shown the ability to use audition effectively.
Oral method (also known as *auditory, verbal-oral,* or *oral-aural*)	Uses audition and speechreading for speech perception
Rochester method (also known as *neo-oralism* or *visible speech*)	Uses fingerspelling to supplement audition and speechreading for speech perception
Cued speech	Uses eight hand shapes and four hand positions (32 cues) to supplement audition and lipreading for speech perception Cues allow homophonous words to be distinguished and clarified.
Manually coded English (also known as *sign systems*)	Reception and expression of language via formal gestures, fingerspelling, signs that represent oral English in manual form, or any combination of these Manual symbols are produced in English word order and can be accompanied by common word endings. Several sign systems have been developed, including Seeing Essential English (SEE$_1$), Signing Exact English (SEE$_2$), and Signed English.
American sign language (also known as *ASL* or *AMESLAN*)	The natural language of the deaf community ASL differs from English at all structural levels, having its own morphology, syntax, and lexicography.
Bilingual-bicultural approach	An educational approach advocated by members of the deaf culture Recognizes ASL as the natural language of the deaf, encourages its use, and teaches oral English, manually coded English, or both as a second language
Total communication (also known as *TC*)	A philosophy, rather than a specific methodology Uses any and all communication methods that prove successful for a particular child In practice, TC programs typically employ the simultaneous use of speech and manually coded English for reception and expression of language.

Methodology	Description
Deaf-blind methods	Uses the tactile reception of speech motor patterns, fingerspelling, or signs
	Speech movements are monitored by placing a hand on the face and neck of the speaker (Tadoma method).
	Fingerspelling and signs are monitored by placing hands on the hands of the sender.

Quantitative scales are available to assist parents and professionals in the selection process. The Deafness Management Quotient uses a weighted assessment of residual hearing, central intactness, intellectual factors, family constellation, and socioeconomic condition to arrive at recommendations regarding oral versus TC placement.[27] The Spoken Language Predictor Index evaluates hearing capacity, aided performance, language competence, nonverbal intelligence, family support, and speech communication attitude to determine the degree to which speech, signs, or both should be emphasized.[28]

Language Assessment and Intervention

The majority of tests designed to evaluate the language abilities of normal-hearing children can be used with the hearing impaired. There are, however, potential shortcomings to this approach. First, there are a limited number of standardized tests that assess the unique language deficits associated with hearing loss. Second, the effects of auditory confusions, speechreading, and short-term memory for signs on test taking ability are not fully understood and can confound the validity of particular instruments to varying degrees.[29] For these reasons, a battery of informal and formal measures should be used to evaluate the language abilities of hearing-impaired children. The specific tests and procedures that are used to assess the language skills of infants and toddlers are described in Chapter 7 and in Appendixes A and B.

Traditional models of language intervention for hearing-impaired children are classified as natural or grammatical. In natural language approaches, remediation parallels the normal developmental sequence of language forms and functions. Language is taught through meaningful experiences in natural and activity-oriented communicative situations. Grammatical approaches focus on the structure of language. Intervention using the grammatical approach consists of formal instruction and drills to establish the appropriate use of syntactic rules and sentence structure.

The selection of a particular method of intervention depends on the child's age, communication style, language skills, educational setting, and degree of hearing loss.[2] Natural approaches are most appropriate for infants and toddlers. They can be used with children who exhibit little or no language ability and are conducive to home-based programming. As the child grows and language skills emerge, formal grammatical techniques can be incorporated into remediation to

Table 9.5 Normal Developmental Sequence of Auditory Skills during the First Year of Life

1. Reflexive: Child responds reflexively to suprathreshold sounds (e.g., startle, initiation or cessation of activity, stirring or arousal from sleep, eye widening or blink, crying).
2. Attending and alerting: Child attends to environmental sounds and voices. Listening attitude, searching behavior, and changes in facial expression may be seen.
3. Localization: Sources of sounds can be identified. Child may turn or move toward sounds.
4. Distance hearing: Infant localizes and attends to sounds at varying distances.
5. Gross environmental discrimination, identification, and comprehension: Child can associate environmental sounds with their sources. May point to, manipulate, or imitate sound sources.
6. Vocal discrimination, identification, and comprehension: Child can discriminate and associate gross vocal sounds, words, and phrases with their sources and meanings.
7. Speech discrimination, identification, and comprehension: Speech sounds can be distinguished and comprehended. Perceptual skills for vowels precede those for consonants.

ameliorate specific language deficits. A more detailed review of language intervention procedures for infants and toddlers is presented in Chapter 8.

Development of Sensory Skills

Auditory Training

Normal-hearing children acquire auditory skills naturally and early in life in response to continuous auditory stimulation. By 6 months of age, hearing babies can attend to speech at conversational levels, localize the source of sounds, recognize differences in vocal tones, and discriminate the various acoustic features of the speech signal. By 1 year of age, they have developed enough auditory and linguistic ability to recognize their names, familiar words, and simple instructions. The normal developmental sequence of auditory skills is shown in Table 9.5.

Hearing loss can prevent or delay the acquisition of auditory skills by depriving a child of auditory stimulation. The effect of hearing impairment on auditory development depends on its severity and time of onset. Children with severe to profound impairments do not acquire auditory skills without amplification and intervention. Hard-of-hearing children can acquire some basic auditory behaviors naturally (e.g., auditory attention, localization), but the development of more sophisticated skills is delayed until amplification is obtained.

The goal of auditory training is to maximize the receptive abilities of hearing-impaired children by developing their listening skills to the fullest extent. Several approaches to auditory training have been developed and include the Carhart method,[30] traditional approaches,[31] the acoupedic method,[32] the cognitive auditory method,[33] and the verbo-tonal method.[34] Each approach is based on the normal developmental sequence of auditory skills, but the approaches differ in their degree of structure, manner of delivery and reinforcement, and use of supplemental sensory devices.

The auditory training of infants and toddlers is most effective when it is conducted during normal daily activities. As a child's skills develop, structured activities can be incorporated into the remediation program to facilitate the growth of advanced auditory functions (e.g., sequential memory, closure, selective attention). Home-based intervention requires the informed participation of family members. They should be familiar with the developmental sequence of auditory behaviors as well as therapeutic techniques and materials. A variety of auditory training programs are available commercially. Many are either written for parents or can be adapted for their use.

Visual Training

Most educational methodologies encourage the use of speechreading to maximize the receptive abilities of hearing-impaired children. Few, however, incorporate structured visual training into the early stages of intervention. As Hipskind[35] explained, "there is a tendency to allow this aspect of rehabilitation to develop naturally in conjunction with the acquisition of auditory, speech, and linguistic skills" (p. 150).

Although visual training is not formalized early in remediation, steps can be taken during this period to maximize the reception of visual linguistic cues. Ophthalmologic testing should be conducted as early as possible. Visual acuity must be within normal limits or corrected to normal limits to enable the reception of the subtle articulatory movements of speech. Speechreading ability is also affected by distance and viewing angle. Perceptual skills are optimal when speech is received at a horizontal viewing angle of 0–45 degrees and from a distance no greater than 10 feet.[36] Proper room illumination must be maintained, and speakers should avoid positioning themselves where light sources cause their faces to be in shadow.

Structured speechreading exercises can be incorporated into remediation as a child's oral language ability develops. Historically, both analytic and synthetic approaches have been used to teach speechreading. Analytic methods concentrate on the visual identification of the individual components of speech (e.g., phonemes, syllables, words). Synthetic methods focus on the comprehension of the general meaning of a message rather than the identification of each component within the message. Most contemporary methods combine these two approaches in their training procedures. An excellent description of the combined approach to speechreading training is presented by Jeffers and Barley.[3]

Speech Training

Speech assessment of hearing-impaired children should focus on three areas of production: suprasegmental skills, segmental skills, and speech intelligibility. Intelligibility testing may not be appropriate for young children with limited speech skills. As a child's expressive ability increases, however, this measure should be incorporated into the assessment battery.

Children must demonstrate the spontaneous and consistent use of voice for communicative purposes before speech skills can be developed. Although an auditory-verbal communication style evolves naturally in most children with mild-to-moderate hearing loss, a concerted effort by parents and clinicians usually is required to sustain the vocal behaviors of children with severe-to-profound impairments. Early vocalizations can be encouraged by involving children in activities that require the frequent use of voice (e.g., verbal play, singing, game playing, imitation of nonspeech sounds). Voice-activated toys and visual devices can also be used to elicit vocal behavior. Any activity that encourages a child to initiate, imitate, or respond to vocalization should be noted and used as a foundation for further training.

Formal speech-training programs use distinctive feature contrasts,[37] word and syllable productions,[38] a hierarchy of segmental and suprasegmental contrasts,[39] or any combination of these to develop the speech skills of hearing-impaired children. Auditory models should be used whenever a child is able to detect and discriminate the acoustic features of the stimulus. Most children, however, require the combined use of auditory, visual, and tactile sensory modalities to acquire and monitor target productions. A variety of techniques can be used to provide supplemental visual and tactile feedback. Electronic and computer-based instruments (e.g., the IBM Speech Viewer II, spectrographic displays, electropalatography, vibrotactile devices) provide detailed visual and tactile feedback for a variety of suprasegmental and segmental characteristics. Simpler, less costly techniques include speechreading, visual prompts and hand cues, and tactile impressions of the breath stream, laryngeal and nasal vibration, and articulator location.

Currently, the Ling approach is the most widely used speech-training program for the hearing impaired.[39] In this method, speech skills are developed systematically at the phonetic and phonologic levels of production. Phonetic training is centered around the acquisition of orosensorimotor patterns at the syllabic level. Children are taught to produce syllabic targets in isolation, in repeated and alternated strings, and with variations in prosody to develop automaticity and coarticulatory ability. The phonologic level of training emphasizes the carryover of phonetic skills to conversational speech.

REFERENCES

1. Peterson GE, Barney HL. Control methods used in a study of the identification of vowels. J Acoust Soc Am 1954;24:183.
2. Davis JM, Hardick EJ. Rehabilitative Audiology for Children and Adults. New York: Macmillan, 1986.
3. Jeffers J, Barley M. Speechreading (Lipreading). Springfield, IL: Thomas, 1971;3.
4. Norlin PF, Van Tasell DJ. Linguistic skills of hearing impaired children. Monogr Contemp Audiol 1980;1:1.
5. Elfenbein JL, Hardin-Jones MA, Davis JM. Oral communication skills of children who are hard of hearing. J Speech Hear Res 1994;37:216.

6. Seyfried DN, Hutchinson JM, Smith LL. Language and Speech of the Hearing Impaired. In RL Schow, MA Nerbonne (eds), Introduction to Aural Rehabilitation (2nd ed). Austin, TX: Pro-Ed 1989;181.
7. Stark RE. Phonatory Development in Young Normally Hearing and Hearing-Impaired Children. In I Hochberg, H Levitt, MJ Osberger (eds), Speech of the Hearing Impaired: Research, Training, and Personnel Preparation. Baltimore: University Park Press, 1983;251.
8. Stoel-Gammon C, Otomo K. Babbling development of hearing-impaired and normally hearing subjects. J Speech Hear Disord 1986;51:33.
9. Tait M, Lutman ME. Comparison of early communicative behavior in young children with cochlear implants and with hearing aids. Ear Hear 1994;15:352.
10. West J, Weber J. A phonological analysis of the spontaneous language of a four-year-old hard-of-hearing child. J Speech Hear Disord 1973;38:25.
11. American Speech-Language-Hearing Association. Preferred practice patterns for the professions of speech-language pathology and audiology: aural rehabilitation. ASHA 1993;35:23.
12. Downs M. The establishment of hearing aid use: a program for parents. MAICO Audiology Library Series 1967;4.
13. Ross M. Hearing Aid Selection for Preverbal Hearing Impaired Children. In M Pollack (ed), Amplification for the Hearing Impaired. New York: Grune & Stratton, 1975;207.
14. Elfenbein JL, Bentler RA, Davis JM, Niebuhr DP. Status of school children's hearing aids relative to monitoring practices. Ear Hear 1988;9:212.
15. Northern JL, Downs MP. Hearing in Children (4th ed). Baltimore: Williams & Wilkins, 1991.
16. Fryauf-Bertschy H. Pediatric cochlear implantation: an update. Am J Audiol 1993;2:13
17. Tyler RS. Cochlear implants and the deaf culture. Am J Audiol 1993;2:26.
18. Fryauf-Bertschy H, Tyler RS, Kelsay DM, Gantz BJ. Performance over time of congenitally and postlingually deafened children using multichannel cochlear implants. J Speech Hear Res 1992;35:913.
19. Dawson PW, Blamey PJ, Rowland LC, et al. Cochlear implants in children, adolescents, and prelinguistically deafened adults: speech perception. J Speech Hear Res 1992;35:401.
20. Dawson PW, Blamey PJ, Dettman SJ, et al. A clinical report on speech production of cochlear implant users. Ear Hear 1995;16:551.
21. Eilers RE, Cobo-Lewis AB, Vergara KC, et al. A longitudinal evaluation of the speech perception capabilities of children using multichannel tactile vocoders. J Speech Hear Res 1996;39:518.
22. Osberger MJ, Maso M, Sam LK. Speech intelligibility of children with cochlear implants, tactile aids, or hearing aids. J Speech Hear Res 1993;36:186.
23. Steffans ML, Eilers RE, Fishman L, et al. Early vocal development in tactually aided children with severe-profound hearing loss. J Speech Hear Res 1994;37:700.
24. Boothroyd A. Special issue: auditory and tactile presentation of voice fundamental frequency as a supplement to speech reading. Ear Hear 1988;9:6.
25. Geers AE, Moog JS. Speech perception and production skills of students with impaired hearing from oral and total communication education settings. J Speech Hear Res 1992;35:1384.
26. Caccamise F, Hatfield N, Brewer L. Manual/simultaneous communication research: results and implications. Am Ann Deaf 1978;123:803.
27. Downs MP. The deafness management quotient. Hearing and Speech News Jan–Feb 1974.
28. Geers AE, Moog JS. Predicting spoken language acquisition of hearing impaired children. J Speech Hear Disord 1987;42:84.

29. Moeller MP, Osberger MJ, Morford JA. Speech-Language Assessment and Intervention with Preschool Hearing-Impaired Children. In JG Alpiner, PA McCarthy (eds), Rehabilitative Audiology: Children and Adults. Baltimore: Williams & Wilkins, 1987;163.
30. Carhart R. Auditory Training. In H Davis, R Silverman (eds), Hearing and Deafness (2nd ed). New York: Holt, Rinehart & Winston, 1960;368.
31. Erber NP. Auditory Training. Washington, DC: Alexander Graham Bell Association for the Deaf, 1982.
32. Pollack D. Educational Audiology for the Limited Hearing Infant. Springfield, IL: Thomas, 1970.
33. Grammatico L. The development of listening skills. Volta Rev 1975;77:303.
34. Guberina P. Studies in the Verbo-Tonal System. Columbus, OH: Ohio State University Press, 1964.
35. Hipskind NM. Visual Stimuli in Communication. In RL Schow, MA Nerbonne (eds), Introduction to Aural Rehabilitation (2nd ed). Austin, TX: Pro-Ed, 1989;125.
36. Caccamise F, Meath-Lang B, Johnson D. Assessment and use of vision: critical needs of hearing-impaired students. Am Ann Deaf 1981;26:361.
37. Bennett C. Articulation training of profoundly hearing-impaired children: a distinctive feature approach. J Commun Disord 1978;11:433.
38. Abraham S, Werner F. Efficacy of word training vs. syllable training on articulatory generalization by severely hearing-impaired children. Volta Rev 1985;87:97.
39. Ling D. Speech and the Hearing Impaired Child: Theory and Practice. Washington, DC: Alexander Graham Bell Association for the Deaf, 1976.

10

Marketing What We Have to Offer

Frances P. Billeaud

Marketing is a constant challenge for communicative disorders specialists. It is a very important facet of the array of professional responsibilities the speech-language pathologist (SLP) assumes, and one in which few university training programs provide instruction. In this era of managed care with its emphasis on reduction of costs, often by restricting the use of specialists, marketing what we have to offer to administrative entities, managed care organizations, and consumer groups is a task for which we must develop skills. Koyanagi and Lorber[1] have provided an excellent set of suggestions and guidelines in this regard in their article, "Can managed care meet the mental health needs of very young children?" Their practical suggestions are applicable across other infant-toddler-family service provision areas.

Marketing does not have to be expensive or glitzy. It must serve the purpose (e.g., promote a new program, increase use of an existing service, educate peer professionals about issues in communicative development and its relationship to their own specialties, or inform parents that early intervention with infants and toddlers is effective). It must meet the needs of the marketer. It must be delivered in a format that is appealing, direct, informative, and accessible to the target audiences. The first task, then, is to identify the audiences and determine how to reach them most efficiently. The next thing to do is to decide what message(s) to deliver: what the audience needs to know, what degree of detail is necessary, and what level of language should be used.

Marketing tools include the SLP's business card; short topic-specific informational sheets, pamphlets, or brochures; cover letters directed to a specific person or group when reports are transmitted; presentations to professional peer groups; displays or programs provided at events such as health fairs; personal visits to key personnel (e.g., administrators, prospective or existing referral sources); and short articles submitted to in-house newsletters, community newspapers, or periodical publications of organizations. Marketing tools also include appearances on television or radio programs to provide information about communicative development in children, how to handle particular disorders, and how to access parent resources.

Organized (as opposed to haphazard) marketing takes time but is an essential part of conducting a professional practice. It can yield benefits that range from improved understanding of the services SLPs offer to increased

197

referrals from professional colleagues, and from increased visibility in the community to improved use of services for infants and toddlers at risk for communication disorders.

More specifically, in keeping with the focus of this book, targeted marketing efforts should be directed at expanding the use of services for infants and toddlers with or at risk for communicative disorders and improving the understanding of the purpose of those services among administrators, peer professionals, and parents. Such efforts can be organized around the services themselves or around the targeted age groups.

MARKETING THE SPEECH-LANGUAGE PATHOLOGIST'S SERVICES FOR NEWBORNS

Rehabilitation units in hospitals usually have SLPs on staff. The same is not true of most neonatal intensive care units (NICUs), although increasing numbers of SLPs are being hired in that environment. An increasing body of literature is available on the advantages of multidisciplinary teams that include the SLP in the NICU. In attempting to establish a presence on such teams, a specialized marketing effort must be implemented with the medical staff and the hospital administration.

Newborns admitted to the NICU are often small, sick, and fragile. Resolution of the health problems is the primary concern of the medical staff. Recognition of that fact assists the SLP who wishes to establish a presence in the NICU and assists in knowing how to approach the marketing effort. Sparks and colleagues[2] suggested that the SLP have a specific plan in mind when meeting with the medical staff to discuss involvement in the NICU: (1) Establish that the clinician has a role on the health care team, (2) explain biological and caregiving conditions that place communication development at risk and how those conditions interact, (3) explain principles of communicative assessment within the context of the developmental assessment process, (4) explain principles of intervention with this population, and (5) introduce prevention as a role for clinicians in the NICU.

Nurse-practitioner Lee McKenzie[3] stressed the importance of approaching the busy NICU staff initially as an interested observer who is there to learn the system. She suggested that the "nontraditional" professional who seeks to be a part of the NICU team should ask for information about caregiving provided by a key staff member (she suggested that it be a nurse). It is important to know the jobs of those who work on the NICU and to stay out of the way as they conduct routine procedures. Showing genuine interest, avoiding violation of professional space, learning the routines and the chain of command, and being a "presence" that becomes recognized on the unit, McKenzie suggested, go a long way toward making the staff receptive to listening to what you have to offer.

Sparks and colleagues[2] echoed this advice: "To participate in the NICU, clinicians must establish credibility by studying medical conditions, gain expertise by working with pediatric patients, and be willing to commit time. It is also advantageous to be able to assist with feeding." The latter, of course, also requires specific training.

If it is difficult to schedule conferences with the staff members of newborn care units, videotaped presentations lasting no more than 10–20 minutes can be a way to reach key personnel. Banigan[4] (1991) has used this technique in working with hospital pediatric staff members for some time. It has also been the author's experience that colleagues in pediatrics, and obstetrics and gynecology departments enjoy having such in-service materials available to them for use in the doctors' lounge during lulls in their schedules or to take home for viewing at a convenient time. Nurses also seem to appreciate the convenience of this approach.

Research should be done by the SLP regarding the hospital's stated position, if any, on what constitutes quality care for all patients. If there is a multi-hospital corporate structure, do other hospitals in the corporate system use SLPs on their NICU staffs? Would inclusion of the SLP on *this* hospital's NICU team be advantageous to the hospital administration in terms of accrediting criteria, community marketing efforts, or attracting desired medical staff personnel?

Preparing a concise proposal for administrative and medical staff review is required at the appropriate time. Supporting information can be included as attachments or exhibits when the proposal is presented for consideration.

MARKETING SERVICES FOR INFANTS AND TODDLERS IN THE COMMUNITY

Not all babies who are at risk for communicative disorders are graduates of NICUs. Many are discharged from well-baby nurseries or are born at home and were never in a hospital nursery. Maternal- and child-health clinics in the public sector or private pediatric practices may be the SLP's first point of contact with these infants and their parents. The communicative disorders specialist who wishes to work with the infant-toddler-family population should be familiar with the federally funded Early and Periodic Screening, Diagnosis, and Testing [EPSDT] program provided by public Maternal and Child Health Services. The EPSDT program is responsible for conducting regular, comprehensive health screenings, including screening for communication problems for children from birth through the school years. Marketing services to the administrators of such programs is advisable. An example of a tool that can be used in such an effort is shown in Table 10.1. Providing multiple copies with a request that they be circulated to the nursing staff is a means of getting information to personnel who work with the population on a daily basis, and the "sampler" could serve as a means of raising the awareness level among nurses about risk identification for communication disorders.

Other community agencies include medical clinics, early-intervention programs, private practices, social-service agencies, preschools and child care centers, and public-health programs. This diversity obviously indicates that marketing efforts must be targeted to the specific entity, its consumer group(s), or both. Knowing the structure of the agency, the composition of its staff, pro-

Table 10.1 A Sampler of Etiologies Associated with Communicative Disorders in Infants and Toddlers

Hearing impairment
    Congenital hearing loss (genetic, syndromes, infections, anomalies)
    Transitory hearing loss (i.e., persistent, chronic episodes of otitis media; viral and bacterial illnesses; noise-induced problems; acute trauma)
    Acquired or adventitious hearing loss
        Iatrogenic (e.g., ototoxic drugs)
        Etiologically traced to illnesses (especially viral infections) or injuries
Delayed or disordered receptive language development
    Mental retardation
    Hearing impairment (see above)
    Other sensory impairments (especially severe vision impairments)
    Metabolic disorders (e.g., phenylketonuria)
    Syndromes not identified with chromosomal anomalies (e.g., fetal alcohol syndrome)
    Psychiatric disorders (e.g., psychopathologies such as autism, pervasive developmental disorder)
    Chromosomal disorders (e.g., fragile X syndrome)
Delayed onset of speech without obvious receptive language impairment
    Structural anomalies (e.g., cleft palate, choanal atresia)
    Neurophysiologic and neurobehavioral organization disorders (e.g., cerebral palsy, oral apraxia, sequelae of prenatal cocaine exposure)
    Environmental factors (e.g., abuse or neglect, unusual child-rearing practices that discourage speech or language development, lack of experience or poor speech models)
    Attention deficit disorder with or without hyperactivity
    Idioglossia (associated with multiple births)
Disordered development of speech or language
    All factors listed in sections above
    Neuropathologies (e.g., brain damage, facial or glossal nerve paralysis)
    Psychopathologies (e.g., autism, schizophrenia, pervasive developmental disorder not otherwise specified, childhood disintegrative disorder)
    Regression or interrupted development (e.g., trauma, degenerative or progressive disease processes)
    Laryngeal pathologies (e.g., vocal cord stridor, laryngeal web, papillomatosis, damage residual to prolonged or repeated intubation, prolonged tracheostomy with resulting paresis of the vocal cords)
    Velopharyngeal incompetence or insufficiency and other structural anomalies of the oral and laryngeal mechanism
    Language-learning disability (novel within the index family)

grammatic goals, mission statements, and administrative philosophy is important to devising a successful marketing effort.

Many SLPs in private practice provide complimentary consultative services to their colleagues in private pediatric, otorhinolaryngology, plastic surgery, neurology, and family practices. It is highly unlikely that those medical practitioners will, on their own, seek information about the roles of SLPs with infants and their families. An excellent list of suggestions for interacting with pediatricians is provided by Richardson,[5] who is a pediatrician and former president of the American Speech-Language-Hearing Association (ASHA).

The role of the SLP or audiologist seems to assume more visibility after the expected age of speech onset is reached (i.e., 12–14 months), possibly because parents voice their own heightened concerns at or around that time. Unfortunately, there are some health care professionals who persist in advising families to wait until the child has reached the age of 3 years before taking steps to determine why speech has not emerged, especially if the child does not exhibit signs of cognitive deficits or physical anomalies.[5-7] It is obvious that we cannot relax our efforts to keep the professional community and parents advised of the importance of communication competence to the child's cognitive, emotional, social, and educational development.

ONGOING MARKETING STRATEGIES

Marketing is a continuous process in which the SLP remains involved over the course of association with an agency or practice. Different goals and objectives are promoted at different times using different marketing tools. Some of the means by which the SLP can communicate effectively with professional colleagues and parent groups about the importance of early attention to communicative development include the following:

- Presentation at team or staff meetings or meetings of parent groups (Seek invitations to targeted groups.)
- Short videotaped presentations prepared for viewing by team members at their convenience
- Distribution of reprints or copies of pertinent articles from professional journals to key associates with an informal note indicating that you think the colleague may be interested in the topic (depending on circumstances, highlighting passages may be appropriate)
- Short articles prepared for in-house newsletters or other publications
- Participation in seminars, workshops, and staff development activities (Be visible to colleagues at professional gatherings of this nature.)
- Following up on your referrals to other specialists by note, letter, phone, or personal visit
- Requesting permission to attend in-service programs put on for colleagues in related fields and then being there (A shared knowledge base is important.)
- Asking for input from colleagues about standards of care or management of a particular condition or problem; valuing their experience and expertise and letting them know that you do
- Acknowledging your awareness of the contributions of practitioners in other disciplines (e.g., Brazelton, Greenspan, Capute and Accardo, and

Shonkoff and colleagues in medicine; outstanding contributors in psychology and other fields)
- Being visible to professional colleagues and community groups; introducing yourself by your professional title; providing your business card to people at appropriate times
- Sending short thank-you notes for professional courtesies; letting your colleagues know you notice and appreciate their assistance, encouragement, and interest

ASHA has developed specific materials to assist practitioners in devising marketing plans and identifying appropriate marketing tools.[8–11] See Appendix C for information on obtaining these publications from ASHA.

CONCLUSION

The first 36 months of life are the child's most critical developmental period. The rapid and interrelated changes that occur across physical, cognitive, social, and behavioral parameters are integral to development of the communication system. The communication system, in turn, facilitates other areas of maturation and growth and is the foundation on which school success relies. Early identification of children with atypical development is essential if the most effective management is to be a possibility.

Clinical experience and research efforts of professionals who represent many disciplines provide a developing body of information that assists in providing appropriate services to affected children and their families. Selected materials from that body of information are provided in the glossary and appendices that follow this chapter, which are designed to serve as a practical clinical reference. They are meant to be both a resource for practitioners and a stimulus for further exploration of the emerging literature of the field. The materials included address the following areas.

- Terminology used in serving pediatric populations (Glossary)
- Selected developmental norms and expectations and assessment materials (Appendix A)
- Infant feeding and oral motor information; intervention materials (Appendix B)
- Administrative references (Appendix C)

REFERENCES

1. Koyanagi C, Lorber M. Can managed care meet the mental health needs of very young children? Infants Young Child 1997;10:38.
2. Sparks SN, Oliver J, Clark MJ, et al. Infants at Risk for Communication Disorders: The Professionals' Role with the New Born. Short course presented at American Speech-Language-Hearing Association Convention, Boston, November 1988.

3. McKenzie L. How to Start a Grassroots Multidisciplinary Neonatal Intervention Team. Presentation at Region IV Interagency Coordinating Council's Multidisciplinary Conference on Handicapped Infants and Toddlers, Lafayette, LA, October 1990.
4. Banigan R. Letter to author, November 29, 1991.
5. Richardson SO. Pediatrics. In RM Haller, N Sheldon (eds), Speech Pathology and Audiology in Medical Settings. New York: Stratton Intercontinental Medical Books, 1976;37.
6. Alt E. Speech delay predictive of later problems [letter to the editor]. Exceptional Parent 1990;20:8.
7. Moon E. Speech delay predictive of later problems [letter to the editor]. Exceptional Parent 1990;20:7.
8. American Speech-Language Hearing Association. Marketing Manual: A Resource Guide. Rockville, MD: ASHA, 1996.
9. American Speech-Language Hearing Association. Physician Education Program Kit. Rockville, MD: ASHA, 1991.
10. American Speech-Language Hearing Association. Speech-Language Pathology Marketing Kit, Person to Person: Making a Difference. Rockville, MD: ASHA, 1991.
11. American Speech-Language Hearing Association. Marketing to Multicultural Audiences Kit (Speech-Language Pathology). Rockville, MD: ASHA, 1992.

A

Appendix: Normal Development and Infant Assessment Tools

Table A.1 Conversion from Pounds and Ounces to Grams

Pounds	Ounces															
	0	1	2	3	4	5	6	7	8	9	10	11	12	13	14	15
0	0	28	57	85	113	142	170	198	227	255	283	312	340	369	397	425
1	454	482	510	539	567	595	624	652	680	709	737	765	794	822	850	879
2	907	936	964	992	1,021	1,049	1,077	1,106	1,134	1,162	1,191	1,219	1,247	1,276	1,304	1,332
3	1,361	1,389	1,417	1,446	1,474	1,503	1,531	1,559	1,588	1,616	1,644	1,673	1,701	1,729	1,758	1,786
4	1,814	1,843	1,871	1,899	1,928	1,956	1,984	2,013	2,041	2,070	2,098	2,126	2,155	2,183	2,211	2,240
5	2,268	2,296	2,325	2,353	2,381	2,410	2,438	2,466	2,495	2,523	2,551	2,580	2,608	2,637	2,665	2,693
6	2,722	2,750	2,778	2,807	2,835	2,863	2,892	2,920	2,948	2,977	3,005	3,033	3,062	3,090	3,118	3,147
7	3,175	3,203	3,232	3,260	3,289	3,317	3,345	3,374	3,402	3,430	3,459	3,487	3,515	3,544	3,572	3,600
8	3,629	3,657	3,685	3,714	3,742	3,770	3,799	3,827	3,856	3,884	3,912	3,941	3,969	3,997	4,026	4,054
9	4,082	4,111	4,139	4,167	4,196	4,224	4,252	4,281	4,309	4,337	4,366	4,394	4,423	4,451	4,479	4,508
10	4,536	4,564	4,593	4,621	4,649	4,678	4,706	4,734	4,763	4,791	4,819	4,848	4,876	4,904	4,933	4,961
11	4,990	5,018	5,046	5,075	5,103	5,131	5,160	5,188	5,216	5,245	5,273	5,301	5,330	5,358	5,386	5,415
12	5,443	5,471	5,500	5,528	5,557	5,585	5,613	5,642	5,670	5,698	5,727	5,755	5,783	5,812	5,840	5,868

Table A.2 The Cranial Nerves

Number	Name	Summary of Function
I	Olfactory	Smell
II	Optic	Vision
III	Oculomotor	Innervation of muscles to move eyeball, pupil, and upper lid
IV	Trochlear	Innervation of superior oblique muscle of eye
V	Trigeminal	Chewing and sensation to face
VI	Abducens	Abduction of eye
VII	Facial	Movement of facial muscles, taste, salivary glands
VIII	(Vestibular) acoustic	Equilibrium and hearing
IX	Glossopharyngeal	Taste, swallowing, elevation of pharynx and larynx, parotid salivary gland, sensation to upper pharynx
X	Vagus	Taste, swallowing, elevation of palate, phonation, parasympathetic outflow to visceral organs
XI	Accessory	Turning of head and shrugging of shoulders
XII	Hypoglossal	Movement of tongue

Source: Reprinted with permission from R Love, W Webb. Neurology for the Speech-Language Pathologist (3rd ed). Boston: Butterworth–Heinemann, 1996;140.

Table A.3 Language and Brain Growth from Birth to 2 Years

Age	Language Milestones	Brain Weight (g)
Birth	Crying	335
3 mos	Cooing and crying	516
6 mos	Babbling	660
9 mos	Voicing intonated jargon	750
12 mos	Approximating first word	925
18 mos	Early naming	1,024
24 mos	Making two-word combinations	1,064

Source: Reprinted with permission from R Love, W Webb. Neurology for the Speech-Language Pathologist (3rd ed). Boston: Butterworth–Heinemann, 1996;257.

Table A.4 Six Major Events in Central Nervous System Maturation, Neural Abnormalities, and Neuropsychological Consequences That Can Occur during Central Nervous System Maturation

Major Events and Time Period (Listed in Sequential Order)	Etiology of Neural Abnormalities	Neuropsychological Consequences*
1. Dorsal induction 18–26 gestation days	Disorders of neural tube closure	Meningomyelocele and anencephaly, profoundly impaired
2. Ventral induction 4–10 gestation weeks	a. Brain fails to make normal cleavage	Holoprosencephaly, seizures, profoundly impaired
	b. Cyst separates cerebellar hemispheres	Mental retardation, other brain anomalies
3. Proliferation of neurons 2–4 gestation months	a. Head size 2–3 SD below mean, arrested cell division, chromosome abnormality	Microcephaly syndromes, mild to moderate mental retardation, possible cleft lip and cleft palate
	b. Early cessation of cell division	Microcephaly, fetal alcohol syndrome, cognitive impairments
4a. Migration of neurons 8 gestation weeks	Bilateral cleft of cerebral hemispheres, all six cortical layers not formed	Schizencephaly, multiple congenital abnormalities, seizures, sensorimotor deficits
4b. Migration of neurons 11–13 gestation weeks	Smooth brain, few gyri, all six cortical layers not formed, neurons in abnormal locations	Lissencephaly, profoundly impaired, seizures, microcephalic, most die in infancy
4c. Migration of neurons 2–5 gestation months	Failure to develop fibers crossing between cerebral hemispheres	Agenesis of corpus callosum, developmentally delayed, seizures
4d. Migration of neurons 4–5 gestation months	Multiple small shallow convolutions on brain surface, neurons in abnormal locations	Polymicrogyria, possible mental retardation and seizure disorder
5. Organization	a. Axon/dendrite damage due to infection, metabolic disorder	Possible sensory loss, motor loss, language deficit
	b. Synaptic loss due to intoxicant	Language deficit

Major Events and Time Period (Listed in Sequential Order)

	Etiology of Neural Abnormalities	Neuropsychological Consequences*
	c. Synaptic aberrance due to systemic disease	Speech deficit
	d. Tissue infarction due to maternal disease	Memory disorder
6. Myelination 6 gestation months to adolescence and beyond	Demyelination due to disease of cerebral white matter	Leukodystrophies, retardation syndromes, global delays in motor development, language disorder

SD = standard deviation.

*Communication, speech, or language disorders and cognitive deficits are associated with the neuropsychological consequence(s).

Source: Reprinted with permission from T Hallett, A Proctor. Maturation of the central nervous system as related to communication and cognitive development. Infants Young Child 1996;8:3. Copyright 1996, Aspen Publishers.

Table A.5 Primitive and Postural Infantile Reflexes of the First Year

Reflex	Response
Asymmetric tonic neck	Infant extends limbs on chin side and flexes on occiput side when turning head.
Symmetric tonic neck	Infant extends arms and flexes legs with head extension.
Positive support	Infant bears weight when balls of feet are stimulated.
Tonic labyrinthine	Infant may retract shoulder and extend neck and trunk with neck flexion. Tongue thrust reflex may occur.
Segmental rolling	Infant may roll trunk and pelvis segmentally with rotation of head or legs.
Galant	Infant arches body when skin of back is stimulated near vertebral column.
Moro's	Infant may adduce arm and move it upward, followed by arm flexion and leg extension and flexion.

Source: Reprinted with permission from R Love, W Webb. Neurology for the Speech-Language Pathologist (3rd ed). Boston: Butterworth–Heinemann, 1996;278.

Table A.6 Infantile Oral Reflexes

Reflex	Stimulus	Age of Appearance	Age of Disappearance
Rooting	Oral area being touched	Birth	3–6 mos
Suckling	Nipple in mouth	Birth	6–12 mos
Swallowing	Bolus of food in pharynx	Birth	Persists
Tongue	Tongue or lips being touched	Birth	12–18 mos
Bite	Pressure on gums	Birth	9–12 mos
Gag	Tongue or pharynx being touched	Birth	Persists

Source: Reprinted with permission from R Love, W Webb. Neurology for the Speech-Language Pathologist (3rd ed). Boston: Butterworth–Heinemann, 1996;288.

Table A.7   Diagnostic Guide*

	Normal Pattern of Language Development	Deviant Pattern of Language Development in the Clinical Population
Rate	Rapid, samples changing every 3 wks	Slow, consecutive samples similar
Jargon	Intermittent, ceases by 27 mos	Predominant feature continuing beyond 30 mos
Echoing	Intermittent, ceases by 29 mos	Predominant feature continuing beyond 36 mos
Single words	Varies by 12–18 mos	Only nouns beyond 24 mos
Nonverbal cues	Primarily on words or word phrases	Consistent for negative or questions beyond 30 mos
Verbal play	Ceases by 29 mos	Continuing beyond 36 mos
Verbal experimentation	Primarily for phrases and constructions	None or limited
Concepts		
Social terms	By 24 mos	None by 30 mos
Body parts	By 22 mos	None by 24 mos
Numbers	By 20 mos	None by 24 mos
Colors	By 35 mos	None by 42 mos
Announcing action	By 25 mos	None by 30 mos
Self-correcting errors	By 36 mos	None by 48 mos
Commands 100 utterances	By 23 mos	Not by 24 mos
Single words as sentences increase	From 18–23 mos	No decrease of single words by 24 mos
Developmental Sentence Scoring (DSS) becomes valid	By 28 mos	Not valid by 30 mos
DSS and mean sentence length (MSL)	Not growing together, illness affecting only MSL	Growing together, illness affecting DSS
Growth of complexity exceeds growth in length	By 36 mos	Not by 42 mos
Half of sentences correct	By 36 mos	Not by 42 mos
Sentence types	Using declaratives, imperatives, interrogatives by 36 mos	Using only declaratives beyond 36 mos
Simple, compound, complex sentences	By 36 mos	Only simple sentences beyond 36 mos
Past tense		
Irregular	By 29 mos	None by 30 mos
Regular	By 34 mos	None by 36 mos
Overgeneralization	By 36 mos	None by 40 mos
Future tense	By 30 mos	None by 30 mos

Table A.7 (continued)

	Normal Pattern of Language Development	Deviant Pattern of Language Development in the Clinical Population
Indefinite pronouns		
It, this, that	By 18 mos	None by 24 mos
One, some, other	By 24 mos	None by 24 mos
Somebody, something	By 36 mos	None by 36 mos
Personal pronouns		
You	By 27 mos	None by 30 mos
They	By 34 mos	None by 42 mos
He, those	By 36 mos	None by 36 mos
We	By 36 mos	None by 42 mos
Verbs		
Can + verb	By 31 mos	None by 36 mos
Are, will, do + verb	By 36 mos	None by 48 mos
Am + verb + *-ing*	By 36 mos	None by 48 mos
Negatives		
Can't, don't used in sentences	By 36 mos	None by 36 mos
Conjunction and connecting objects and sentences	By 36 mos	None by 36 mos
Questions		
Who? what? where?	By 27 mos	None by 30 mos
Where + subject + *-ing*	By 36 mos	None by 36 mos
What + subject + *-ing*	By 36 mos	None by 42 mos

*The normal pattern column gives the upper age limit of the normal range; the deviant pattern column indicates strikingly different patterns characteristic of language-impaired children.
Source: Reprinted with permission from CR Trantham, JK Pederson. Normal Language Development: The Key to Diagnosis and Therapy for Language-Disordered Children. Baltimore: Williams & Wilkins, 1976;33.

Table A.8   Pragmatic Development in Infants and Toddlers

0–12 Months	1–2 Years	2–3 Years
1. Attempts to imitate the gestures and vocalizations of adults.	1. Uses nonverbal communication to signify intent:	1. Ideational options—learning to express own experience of the phenomena of the external world and the internal world of own consciousness. Learns to be an observer. Begins to use language as a way of talking about the real world.
2. Uses vocalizations in play for self-amusement.	To request (reaching toward the object) To draw attention to object (pointing, showing)	
3. Uses telegraphic devices (rising intonation, vocalization with specifications of desires, negating, imperatives, interrogatives) accompanied by gestures and intonation markers.	To draw attention to self (vocalizing) To request transfer (reaching toward another person)	2. Interpersonal communication. Begins to participate in conversational situations. Learns to adopt a role to express opinions and personality. Dialogue begins.
4. Uses onomatopoetic speech (words that sound like the object to mean the object).	To show dislike (falling tone [intonational pattern]) To show disappearance (slapping or waving)	3. Can make what he or she says operational in the communicative context.
5. Uses perlocutionary behaviors—signals issued by one person that have an affect on the listener that is not necessarily intended (e.g., crying, laughing).	To show rejection (negative head shake) To indicate pleasure (surprise, recognition, smile)	4. Begins to use definite versus indefinite articles (i.e., *the* versus *a* or *an*). Often uses *the* incorrectly. Assumes the listener knows what he or she is talking about.
6. Crying takes on different meanings; is directive for parent and later for child (angry, hungry, cranky). Used to communicate events and needs of infant.	2. Performatives emerge—child uses language with communicative intent. The child may know what is wanted, but the meaning is not necessarily clear to the listener.	5. Can judge quality of language 50% of the time (e.g., polite versus impolite). Does not use consistently.
7. Uses illocutionary behavior—signals to carry out some socially organized action (i.e., intentional communication).	3. Presuppositions also emerge—common shared information regardless of phonetic information; child uses expressions that have shared meaning to both speaker and listener.	6. Uses more action identity tags (e.g., "bow wow," "meow," "choo-choo").
8. Picks up an object and shows it (nonverbal).	4. Begins talking about the inanimate world.	
9. Uses pointing to pick things out and to obtain someone's attention.		
10. Uses gestures communicatively and starts		

Table A.8 (continued)

0–12 Months	1–2 Years	2–3 Years
to perceive reactions (making sure listener is attentive before continuing). 11. Responds to pointing as a communicative gesture (looks in direction adult is pointing instead of focusing on that individual's face or hand). 12. Uses pointing to learn new vocabulary—people in the environment label things for the child. 13. Realizes vocalizations of intonation and articulation have meaning for adults, so borrows some of their sounds ("mama," "dada") and makes up own meanings for vocalizations that have content and expression. 14. Nonverbal vocalizations have functions— (1) instrumental "I want" (satisfies personal needs), (2) regulatory "Do it" (seeks to control behaviors of others)—interactional, personal, heuristic, imaginative.	5. Use of early words to signify communicative intent: Requesting ("milk") Possession ("mine") Imperatives ("up") Problems ("hurt") Statements ("shoe") Give objects ("gimme") Locations ("there") Desires ("I want") 6. At one-word stage—expresses only what is new to child. At two-word stage—expresses new information and given information (uses vocal stress to tell which is which). 7. Vocabulary—transition from own language to adult language; learns that certain sounds have certain meanings. 8. Dialogue—acquires a grammatical structure; can be both speaker and listener; learns some rules of discourse ("when someone talks, you should listen"). 9. Uses increasing tone in inflectional pattern. 10. Literally interprets the things heard; cannot play with words.	7. Some role playing is possible. Takes caregiver's place (e.g., if the mother says, "I can't," the child says, "yes, you can"). 8. Repetition used for: Answering questions (e.g., Do you want milk? "Milk.") Commenting (e.g., We're having hot dogs. "Hot dogs.") Affirming (e.g., We're building a fire. "Oh, go build fire.") Self-informing (e.g., We're cooking sausages. "Cook sausages.") Querying (e.g., Put that on top. "On top?") Imitating (e.g., Hi. "Hi." I'm a good cook. Yes, the greatest. "The greatest.") Reversing directions of an order (e.g., You do it. "No, you do it.") Reversing directions of an information question (e.g., Where's the spoon? "Mommy, where's the spoon?") Clarifying an utterance (e.g., Fab. "Fab, what you mean?")

0–12 Months	1–2 Years	2–3 Years
	11. Verbal turn taking.	9. Acquires morphemes. Uses concepts of past and present inconsistently.
	12. Functions: mathetic, pragmatic, informative.	10. At two-word stage: Word combinations are used to express these functions:
		Identification (e.g., "See doggie.")
		Location (e.g., "Book there.")
		Repetition (see above)
		Nonexistence (e.g., "All gone thing.")
		Negation (e.g., "Not wolf.")
		Possession (e.g., "My candy.")
		Attribution (e.g., "Big car.")
		Question (e.g., "Where ball?")
		11. Functions: ideation, interpersoal, textual.

Source: Adapted with permission from BB Shulman. Pragmatic Development Chart. Mobile, AL: Author, 1991.

Table A.9   References for Infant Feeding, Sucking, and Swallowing Problems

Candidates for feeding assessment are infants who meet identified high-risk criteria. The criteria listed here are those used at the Mapleton Center in Boulder, CO. They were developed by Beth Landry as part of the Neonatal Assessment of Feeding and State Organization.

High-Risk Criteria

Prematurity (≤26 wks)
Small for gestational age
Apgar of less than 7 at 5 mins
Seizures
Sepsis or meningitis
Phototherapy or transfusion
Ventilator therapy
Prolonged hypotonia or hypertonia beyond 24 hrs
Recurrent apnea
Congenital anomalies
Congenital or perinatal infections
Poor endurance for feeding
Abnormal or poor suck
Fussy, overstimulated, or disorganized baby
Drug or alcohol abuse (maternal)
Post extracorporeal mechanical oxygenation
5–7% loss of birth weight

Sequence for Assessment

Gather birth history.
Handle infant to assess tone.
Elicit oral reflexes.
Assess nonnutritive suck.
Apply intervention techniques to establish the best possible performance in all areas.
Gather information from parents.
    Is this a typical feeding?
    What is the child's feeding usually like?
    Is the child gaining weight appropriately?
    How long does a feeding usually take?
    How much does the child usually eat at one feeding?
    How does the child deal with solid foods?
    What is the child's sleep and awake pattern like?

Neonatal Assessment for Feeding and State Organization

Name: _____   Parent or guardian: _____

DOB: _____   Date of initial assessment: _____

Chronological age: _____

Corrected age: _____

Apgar: 1_____   2_____

O$_2$: _____

Weight: _____

Significant medical history

Course of feeding

IV: _____

Gavage: _____   How often? _____

Breast: _____

Bottle: _____   Nipple used: ___ _____

Receiving therapeutic treatment? _____

Oral Reflexes

Reflex	Method to Elicit	Pass	Fail
Root open	Stroke front of lips.	Mouth opens or suck begins.	No opening or suck is seen.
Root open and turn (integrated at 3 mos)	Stroke side of cheek.	Head turns to side stroked, and mouth opens with or without suck.	No head turning and no open or suck is seen.
Suck initiation	Place finger in mouth.	Suck begins strong and immediate.	No suck is initiated, or suck is weak.
Swallow	Give small amount of milk or observe during feeding.	Swallow is immediate after three to four sucks.	Swallow is not seen after seven or more sucks.
Hand to mouth	Observe child.	Hand to mouth is seen purposively without assistance or wrapping.	Hand to mouth is not seen.
Bite	Place finger in mouth.	No bite is felt.	Bite is felt.
Gag	Observe during above procedures and during feed.	Gag is not observed, or a weak gag may be seen.	Gag is observed.

Table A.9 (continued)

Techniques to Improve Oral Motor Function

Techniques to facilitate oral reflexes

To reduce bite:

 Rub gums in four quadrants; wait for swallow.

To reduce gag:

 Use firm pressure when touching.

 Massage cheeks in small circles.

 Use finger and place some milk in buccal pocket then massage cheek.

 Rub gums with milk on finger or nipple.

 Gradually and firmly stroke the tongue from back to front at midline.

 "Walk" back on tongue.

To improve root and open:

 Touch lip with bottle, nipple, or finger and give a long pause to allow mouth to open.

 Place small amount of fluid on lip and wait for open and possibly suck.

 Press firmly in the palm of the baby's hand (palmomental reflex).

To increase hand to mouth:

 Swaddle infant.

 Keep infant's shoulders and arms rolled forward.

 Assist hand to mouth to console baby.

Techniques to improve jaw control and movement

 Stroke massage forward from back of jaw to front.

 Apply quick, firm taps under chin.

 Flexed body position.

 Give jaw stabilization when feeding by placing finger under jaw.

Techniques to improve normal tongue position and movement

 Stroke tongue from back to front at midline and sides.

 "Walk" back on tongue.

 Let baby suck on your finger when non-nutritive sucking; if tongue is humped, apply firm pressure to midtongue blade.

 To continue tongue movement, apply firm strokes under chin and move finger back to front.

Techniques to improve lip movement

 Massage cheeks and lips.

 Snap lips.

 Lip flicks.

 Hold cheeks and pull forward with nippling.

 Give jaw support.

 Keep the infant's head flexed forward and chin tucked.

Techniques to Improve Coordination

Use tongue, jaw, and lip techniques.

Reduce all external stimulation.

If the child is 3–4 mos or older, provide a distraction, especially if initiation is difficult (e.g., television, music, toy).

Provide rhythm with movement.

Determine the baby's rhythm and try to impose a rhythm depending on skill level.

Pump the bottle then pause, remove the bottle or tip it back until the baby swallows.

Allow pauses when the infant is panting, disorganized, or fatigued.

Impose pauses in the feed as above.

Try a Haberman feeder if swallow is good, but suck is poor due to initiation, suction, or expression difficulties.

Experiment with a variety of nipples. Give a preemie nipple if weak suck and fatigue are factors.

A cardiac baby may nipple better when positioned in more extension.

Hold baby at an incline of less than 45 degrees.

Source: Reprinted with permission from MB Landry. Neonatal Assessment of Feeding and State Organization. Boulder, CO: NAFSO, 1990.

Table A.10 Oral-Motor and Swallow Assessment and Intervention for Infants with Craniofacial Anomalies

All neonates have two basic needs to sustain life: respiration and nutrition. An interdisciplinary team is needed to deal with the complex issues presented by infants with craniofacial anomalies. The speech-language pathologist (SLP) has a major role on the team as decisions are made regarding management of oral-motor function, which underlies later speech development. The SLP's role also includes contributing information and guidance regarding early communicative development, much of which occurs during the infant's feedings. The outline below highlights issues that must be addressed in providing appropriate care to infants who have craniofacial anomalies.

I. Interdisciplinary team for feeding
   A. Neonatologist: overall status
   B. Otolaryngologist: airway
   C. Nutritionist: dietary issues
   D. SLP: oral-motor function and communication
   E. Occupational therapist: positioning and tone
   F. Nursing: primary feeding
   G. Maxillofacial: consideration of prosthesis
   H. Social worker: family issues
II. Assessment
   A. Tone (overall and oral-motor)
   B. Cleft
   C. Neurologic status (i.e., alertness)
   D. Communication and bonding
   E. Structure (e.g., tracheoesophageal fistula)
III. Oral-motor assessment
   A. Lips, mandible, tongue, and palate for symmetry, strength, and coordination
   B. Cleft factors: width, length, location, surrounding structures, and tissues
   C. Oral-motor function correlated with anatomy
      1. Generation of negative intraoral pressure
      2. Movement against nipple
      3. Deficits matched to feeding devices
IV. Oral feeding guidelines (stable airway and neurologically normal)
   A. Upright position
   B. Haberman feeder (Medela, Inc., P.O. Box 386, Crystal Lake, IL 60014; phone: [800] 435-8316), which allows infant or feeder to control flow of milk with a specially designed valving system.
   C. Large X-cut nipple with careful placement
   D. Frequent burping
   E. Small frequent feedings (i.e., 30 mins maximum)
   F. Applying external pressure to cheeks and mandible
   G. Rule of thumb for quantity at 1–2 wks of age: 30 cc (3 oz)/lb per day
V. Breast feeding with cleft
   A. Isolated cleft lip: some success
   B. Isolated cleft palate: usually difficult
   C. Complete cleft lip and palate: very difficult

VI. Palatal feeding prostheses
    A. Indications
        1. Large bilateral cleft lip and palate
        2. Insufficient seal with nipple
        3. Feeding problems for longer than 2–3 wks
    B. Purposes[a]
        1. Aid in deglutition
        2. Aid in correct tongue position
        3. Enhance sucking pattern
        4. Prevent collapse of arches
        5. Ease burden on nursing staff
    C. Precautions
        1. Irritation of mucous membrane
        2. Edema of mucous membrane
        3. Not an aid in preventing otitis media
        4. Replacement needed with growth
        5. Oral hygiene
VII. Nonoral feeders
    A. Airway compromise (Robin malformation sequence)
        1. *U*-shaped palatal cleft
        2. Micrognathia
        3. Glossoptosis
        4. Upper-airway obstruction
    B. Prematurity (low birth weight with neurologic impairment)
        1. Depressed sucking reflex
        2. Weak suck (trisomy 21 syndrome, Möbius' sequence, Arnold-Chiari malformation, clefting)
        3. Uncoordinated suck (central nervous system asphyxia, Arnold-Chiari malformation)
VIII. Types of nonoral feeding
    A. Orogastric feeding
    B. Nasogastric feeding
    C. Gastrostomy
IX. Treatment for nonoral feeders
    A. Oral-motor stimulation
        1. Stroking rhythmically
        2. Nonnutritive sucking
    B. Goals with tube feeders[b]
        1. Improved postural control
        2. Improved pharyngeal airway control
        3. Touch and movement used communicatively
        4. Response to normalization
        5. Rhythmic suck, swallow, and respiratory pattern
        6. Reduction of gastroesophageal reflux
        7. Improved tone and movement in face
        8. Use of lips and tongue to explore environment
        9. Sound-play facilitation
      10. Total communication approach in learning environment

Table A.10 (continued)

X. Feeding in the postoperative period
  A. Lip surgery
     1. Cup into side of mouth away from cleft
     2. Syringe with soft tubing
     3. Breast feeding[c]
  B. Palate surgery
     1. Cup feeding (duration variable per surgeon)
     2. No chewable food
     3. No pacifiers, straws, spoons, forks, or "tippy" cups
  C. Sequence for texture changes
     1. First 4–6 mos: formula
     2. Between 4 and 6 mos: strained baby food
     3. 10–11 mos: lumpy foods (these are more difficult to introduce if delayed to 14–16 mos)

[a]Finger IM, Guerra LR. Provisional restoration in maxillofacial prosthetics. Dental Clinics of North America 1989;3:435.
[b]Morris S, Klein MD. Prefeeding Skills. Austin, TX: Pro-Ed, 1987.
[c]Weatherly-White RCA. Surgical Timing and Postoperative Feeding in the Cleft-Lip Child. In DA Kernahan, SW Rosenstein (eds), Cleft Lip and Palate: A System of Management. Baltimore: Williams & Wilkins, 1990.
Note: See also Wolf LS, Glass RP. Feeding and Swallowing Disorders in Infancy: Assessment and Management. Tucson, AZ: Communication Skill Builders, 1992.
Source: Reprinted with permission from JC Arvedson. Presentation given at the 1990 ASHA Convention, Seattle, November 1990.

Name of child:_____ DOB:_____

Gestational age at birth:_____ Birth weight:____g *or* ____lbs ____oz
Where delivered?_____ Apgar at 1 min: _____ 5 min_____
By whom delivered?_____ Birth order in family:_____
Type delivery: Vgn____ C-sec____ Brch____ Ftlng____ Stargaze____
            Multiple____ (# of sibs____) Other____
List known complications:_____

Parent(s) name(s):_____
_____Natural _____Adoptive _____Foster
Mailing address:_____
Home address:_____
Phone:_____(H) _____(Mo.B) _____(Fr.B)
Child's present physician(s):_____ Address:_____

Name and position of person completing this form:_____
Who referred child/family here?_____
Services being requested:_____

Did mother receive regular prenatal care? ____Y ____N

Potential Risk Factor Checklist

Verify presence or absence of every item. Enter annotations for any "yes" item; provide specifics from interview, medical records, or both; attach information to this form as necessary.

Maternal factors	Yes	No	Annotations
Previous preterm births	___	___	_____
Repeated miscarriages	___	___	_____
Miscarriage adjacent to this pregnancy	___	___	_____
Stillbirth(s)	___	___	_____
Unexplained fetal or neonatal deaths (e.g., sudden infant death syndrome)	___	___	_____
Cervical incompetence	___	___	_____
Placental abnormalities	___	___	_____
Genetic disease or chromosomal disorders	___	___	_____
Infections in first trimester	___	___	_____
Blood group problems (i.e., Rh incompatibility)	___	___	_____
Toxemia of pregnancy	___	___	_____
Unexplained bleeding	___	___	_____
Significantly high or low blood pressure	___	___	_____
Maternal diabetes	___	___	_____

Figure A.1 Risk history: long form by Frances P. Billeaud, M.A., CCC/SLP. (Duplicated with permission from the Louisiana Region II Interagency Coordinating Council Multidisciplinary Evaluation Project, Baton Rouge, LA, 1992.)

Maternal seizures   ___   ___
Medications, drugs, or alcohol   ___   ___   Please specify: _____
Other conditions   ___   ___   What and when: _____

Labor, delivery, and perinatal factors	Yes	No	Annotations
Abnormal length of pregnancy	___	___	Term: _____
Long or short labor	___	___	Length: _____
Instruments used at delivery	___	___	
Low birth weight (LBW) or very low birth weight (VLBW)	___	___	<2,500 g ___ <1,500 g ___ <1,000 g ___
Intrauterine growth retardation	___	___	
Hyperbilirubinemia (jaundice)	___	___	
Meconium staining or aspiration	___	___	
Central nervous system disorders	___	___	
Abnormal muscle tone	___	___	Hypotonicity ___ Hypertonicity ___ Asymmetry ___
Breathing problems	___	___	Hypoxia ___ Anoxia ___ Cyanosis ___
Oxygen supplement	___	___	For how long? _____
Abnormal head size	___	___	Macrocephaly ___ Microcephaly ___ Asymmetry ___
Convulsions	___	___	When: ___ Type:___
Apnea	___	___	
Excessive irritability	___	___	
Abnormal reflex patterns	___	___	
Respiratory distress	___	___	Bronchopulmonary dysplasia ___ Other ___
Gastrointestinal problems	___	___	
Poor sucking and swallowing	___	___	
Orogastric or nasogastric feeding	___	___	
Poor weight gain (e.g., failure to thrive)	___	___	
Neonatal infections (e.g., human immunodeficiency virus, cytomegalovirus, sepsis, TORCH)	___	___	What: _____
Generalized edema	___	___	
Intracranial hemorrhage	___	___	Grade III ___ Grade IV ___
Congenital anomalies	___	___	What: _____
NICU admission?	___	___	Length of stay: _____
Postnatal drug exposure	___	___	To what? _____
Medications administered	___	___	Specify: _____
Surgeries performed	___	___	Specify: _____
Other conditions and observations worthy of note	___	___	Specify: _____

Developmental factors	Yes	No	Annotations
Serious illnesses	___	___	What: ___ When: _____
Serious trauma or injury	___	___	What: ___ When: _____
Inattention to sounds	___	___	At what age? ___
Known ear infections	___	___	When: ___ Treatment: _____

Figure A.1 (continued)

	Yes	No	
Inattention to visual stimuli	___	___	At what age? ___
Known visual impairment	___	___	Age diagnosed: ___ Type: ___

Delayed pattern of development relating to specific factors

	Yes	No	Annotations
Motor skills	___	___	_____
Social skills	___	___	_____
Speech and language skills	___	___	_____
Adaptive behavior	___	___	_____
Failure to thrive	___	___	_____
Clinical manifestation of undiagnosed anomaly?	___	___	_____
Sleep disturbances	___	___	_____
Eating, chewing, or swallowing disorders	___	___	_____

Other factors

	Yes	No	Annotations
Family hospitalized for genetic or educational problems (e.g., learning disability, reading problems, mental retardation.)	___	___	Specify: _____
Exposure to environmental hazards (e.g., metals, toxic fumes)	___	___	_____
Handicapped sibling	___	___	_____
Other handicapped relatives	___	___	_____
Known allergies	___	___	_____
Physical abuse or neglect	___	___	

Psychosocial factors

	Yes	No	Annotations
Low family income	___	___	_____
Educational level of mother	___	___	Last grade completed: ___
Emotional abuse or neglect	___	___	_____
Little or no opportunity for stimulation	___	___	_____
Low intelligence	___	___	_____
Speech or language impairment	___	___	_____
Vision impairment	___	___	_____
Other (list):	___	___	_____

Other comments and observations to be considered:

_____

_____

_____

_____

List other pertinent reports received:

_____

_____

_____

List other pertinent reports to be obtained and from whom:

_____

_____

_____

_____

Child's name: _____ DOB: _____ Date of evaluation: _____
Parent(s) name(s): _____ Birth weight: _____g Gestational age: _____
Address: _____ Phone: _____
Hospital family service coordinator: _____
School system contact: _____
Primary medical provider (after hospital discharge): _____

_____ meets criteria for services under Part H of the Infant and Toddler
   (child's name)   Act due to the following:

Criteria A
Established medical condition
  ___ Genetic disorder
     Specify: _____
  ___ Congenital or neonatal
     infections or infections
     with a high probability of
     resulting developmental delay
     Specify: _____
  ___ Sensory impairment
     Specify: _____

Developmental
Screening done in neonatal intensive care unit

Screening	Date	Results
PKU	___	_____
T$_4$/TSH (thyroid profile)	___	_____
Hbg. Elect	___	_____
Vision	___	_____
Cranial	___	_____
Ultrasound	___	_____

Criteria B
Biologically at risk
  ___ Birth weight <1,000 g
  ___ Birth weight <1,250 g
     with complicating factors
     requiring level III neonatal
     intensive care unit care
  ___ Hypoxic ischemic
     encephalopathy
  ___ Intraventricular hemorrhage
     grade III or IV or periventric-
     ular leukomalacia
  ___ Technology dependence that
     is likely to result in later
     developmental delay
  ___ Exposure to known teratogens
     or drugs and findings on effects
  ___ Chronic or degenerative
     orthopedic conditions, neuro-
     logic conditions, or both that
     have a high probability of
     developmental delays
     Specify: _____

Status of child's developmental functioning in the following areas: physical status (i.e., motor, vision, and hearing), cognitive, language and speech, self-help:

_____
_____
_____
_____
_____

Identification of Family's and Child's Strengths and Needs

Family's strengths as related to enhancing child's development:

_____
_____
_____

Figure A.2   Hospital-based multidisciplinary evaluation. (Duplicated with permission from the Louisiana Region II Interagency Coordinating Council Multidisciplinary Evaluation Project, Baton Rouge, LA, 1992.)

Family's needs as related to enhancing child's development:

_____
_____
_____
_____

Child's needs:

_____
_____
_____
_____

Individualized Family Service Plan Considerations

_____ Family service coordinator
_____ Early interventionist
_____ Counseling
_____ Nutritionist
_____ Diagnostic and programmatic assessment
_____ Referral to: _____
_____ Other: _____

_____
_____
_____

Additional Comments

_____
_____
_____
_____

Evaluation Participants

_____   _____
Parent(s)   Physician

_____   _____
Social worker   Nurse

_____   _____
Other   Other

Hospital-to-Home Discharge Planning: Individual Family Service Plan

Child's medical needs

Pediatrician:	Ophthalmologist:

Cardiologist:

Neurologist:

Audiologist:

Orthopedist:

Pediatric surgeon:

Geneticist:

Home health:

Lab follow-up:

Home monitoring:

Respiratory support:

Child's educational needs

Nutritional consultation:

Occupational therapy:

Physical therapy:

Speech therapy:

Developmental assessment:

Educational programming:

Figure A.2 (continued)

Discharge planning participants
The following participated in this individualized family service plan:

Signature	*Title*	*Agency*	*Date*

Family needs	**Date**	**Person responsible**
___ Family service coordinator		
___ Community service information		
___ Parent training		
___ Transportation		
___ Financial		
___ Other needs		

Special instructions:

B

Appendix: Assessment and Intervention Tools and Procedures

Table B.1 Expanded List of Tools for Assessment of Early Communication Skills (See Table 7.4 for basic list of assessment tools.)

Instrument	Reference	Features	Recommended Age Group
Assessment of Preterm Infant Behaviors (APIB)	1	APIB was initially designed to be the downward extension of the Neonatal Behavioral Assessment Scale and requires training to administer appropriately.	APIB is used to assess behaviors of premature infants in the hospital setting.
Battelle Developmental Inventory (BDI)	12	BDI uses observation, structured interaction, and caregiver interviews to determine the child's developmental levels across many developmental domains, including communication.	Birth–8 yrs
Bayley Scales of Infant Development	2	This assessment tool compares behaviors of newborns with norms derived from scores of normally developing age peers. It is recommended for infants without known anomalies.	2–30 mos

Table B.1 (continued)

Instrument	Reference	Features	Recommended Age Group
Clinical Linguistic and Auditory Milestones Scale (CLAMS)	6	The format is similar to a physician's standard growth chart. CLAMS is designed for use by physicians during child's office visits with parent acting as informant. CLAMS follows trajectories of communication skill development. The profile indicates whether the child is meeting expected milestones or is lagging behind and in need of referral for assessment.	Birth–24 mos
Denver Developmental Screening Test–II	8	This assessment tool requires administration by a certified examiner or supervision by a certified examiner. Criterion-referenced items assess development across modalities, including communication.	2 wks–6 yrs
Early Language Milestones	7	This assessment tool uses parent report, observation, and elicitation of behaviors to assess level of communicative development (receptive and expressive).	Birth through 3 yrs
Hawaii Early Learning Profile	9	This assessment tool compares infant developmental skills with those expected of age peers and covers a variety of developmental areas, including communication.	Birth through 3 yrs
Neonatal Behavioral Assessment Scale (2nd ed) (NBAS)	3	A trained examiner is required to administer this infant behavior assessment tool. NBAS uses case history and elicited responses to physical and sensory stimuli, along with evaluation of infant state and neurologic status, to determine the child's status.	Appropriate only for newborn, full-term infants.

Instrument	Reference	Features	Recommended Age Group
Receptive Emergent Expressive Language–2 (REEL-2)	4	This screening tool uses parent report to gauge the child's expressive language skills and follows the format of the Vineland Social Maturity Scale.	1 mo–3 yrs
Reynell Developmental Language Scales	13	This assessment tool uses observation, picture and object identification, and object manipulation to assess language abilities.	1–6 yrs
Sequenced Inventory of Communicative Development	10	This assessment tool uses parent report, picture and object identification, and object manipulation to evaluate the child's communicative skills.	4 mos–4 yrs
Southern California Ordinal Scales of Development	5	Separate scales assess various aspects of child development. The Developmental Scale of Communication comprises one unit.	Recommended ages are not specified.
Test of Early Language Development–2 (TELD-2)	11	TELD 2 evaluates receptive and expressive language abilities, including content of language and word forms. It employs a one-to-one situation that presumes child's ability to engage in joint attention and ability to follow simple directions.	2.00–7.11 yrs

References:
1. Als H, Lester BM, Tronik E, Brazelton TB. Assessment of Preterm Infant Behavior (APIB). In HE Fitzgerald, BM Lester, and MW Yogman (eds), Theory and Research in Behavioral Pediatrics (Vol. 1). New York: Plenum, 1982;233.
2. Bayley N. Bayley Scales of Infant Development. San Antonio, TX: The Psychological Corporation, 1993.
3. Brazelton TB. Neonatal Behavioral Assessment Scale (NBAS). White Plains, NY: March of Dimes Materials and Supplies Division, 1984.
4. Bzoch KR, League R. Receptive Expressive Emergent Language Test (REEL) (2nd ed). Austin, TX: Pro-Ed, 1991.
5. California State Department of Education and Diagnostic School for Neurologically Handicapped Children. Southern California Ordinal Scales of Infant Development. Sacramento, CA: Foreworks, 1984.
6. Capute A, Accardo PJ. Clinical Linguistic and Auditory Milestone Scale (CLAMS). Clin Pediatr 1978;17:847.
7. Coplan J. Early Language Milestone Scale (ELM). Tulsa, OK: Modern Education Corporation, 1984.

8. Frankenberg WK, Dodds JB. Denver Developmental Screening II (Denver II). Denver: Ladaca Project and Publishing Foundation, 1990.
9. Furono S, O'Rilley K, Inatsuka T. Hawaii Early Learning Profile (HELP). Palo Alto, CA: Vort Corporation, 1987.
10. Hedrick DL, Prather EM, and Tobin AR. Sequenced Inventory of Communicative Development (SICD). Los Angeles: Western Psychological Corporation, 1984.
11. Hresko WP, Reid DK, and Hammill DD. Test of Early Language Development (TELD-2) (2nd ed). Austin, TX: Pro-Ed, 1991.
12. Newborg J, Stock J, Wnek L. Battelle Developmental Inventory. Allen, TX: DLM/Teaching Resources, 1984.
13. Reynell JK, Gruber CP. Reynell Developmental Language Scales. Los Angeles: Western Psychological Services, 1969.

	Crying	Aggression	Tantrums/Self-Injury	Passive Gaze	Proximity	Pulling Other's Hands	Touching/Moving Other's	Face	Grabs/Reaches	Enactment	Removes Self/Walks Away	Focalization/Noise	Active Gaze	Gives Object	Gestures/Pointing	Facial Expression	Shakes "No"/Nods "Yes"	Intonation	Inappropriate Echolalia	Appropriate Echolalia	One-Word Speech	One-Word Signs	Complex Speech
Requests for affection and interaction. What if child wants:																							
Adult to sit near?																							
Peer to sit near?																							
Adult to look at him or her?																							
Adult to tickle him or her?																							
To be cuddled or embraced?																							
To sit on adult's lap?																							
Other bids for interaction?																							
Requests for adult action. What if child wants:																							
Help with dressing?																							
To be read a book?																							
To play ball or a game?																							
To go outside?																							
To go to a specific place?																							
Other?																							
Requests for object, food, or things. What if child wants:																							
An out-of-reach object?																							
A door or container opened?																							
A favorite food?																							
To turn on music, radio, or TV?																							
To have keys, toys, or a book?																							
Other?																							
Protest. What if:																							
A common routine is dropped?																							

Figure B.1 Cue questions to assess communicative intents and functions. (Reprinted with permission from S Schuler, CA Peck, C Willard, K Theimer. Assessment of communicative means and functions through interview: assessing the communicative abilities of individuals with limited language. Semin Speech Lang 1989;10:51.)

	Crying	Aggression	Tantrums/Self-Injury	Passive Gaze	Proximity	Pulling Other's Hands	Touching/Moving Other's Face	Grabs/Reaches	Enactment	Removes Self/Walks Away	Vocalization/Noise	Active Gaze	Gives Object	Gestures/Pointing	Facial Expression	Shakes "No"/Nods "Yes"	Intonation	Inappropriate Echolalia	Appropriate Echolalia	One-Word Speech	One-Word Signs	Complex Speech	Complex Signs
A favorite food or toy is taken away?																							
The child is taken for a ride without having a desire to do so?																							
Adult terminates interaction?																							
Child is required to do something he or she does not want to do?																							
Declaration or comment. What if child wants:																							
To show you something?																							
To tell you about something?																							
Other?																							

Figure B.1 (continued)

Table B.2 Identifying Areas of Child Competency and Difficulty

Infant Abilities	Parent Abilities	Components of the Interaction
Responsiveness	Parents' awareness of the	Predominant affect
Signaling	child's development	Affectional change
Communication	Parents' ability to function	Initiation of interaction
Cognitive	in the larger environment	Continuation of interaction
Motor	Level of parenting skills	Contingent responsiveness
Emotional	Meaning of the disabling	Pace
Social	condition to the parents	Turn taking
Temperament	and parents' ability to	Use of communicative modalities
Appearance	understand the condition	

ASSESSMENT FRAMEWORK FOR PARENTS AND PROFESSIONALS*

Hanson and Krentz (1986) outlined a method for assisting parents to identify and describe their child's areas of competency and difficulties. Together, parents and professionals review videotaped interactions of the parent and child during teaching, feeding, and play situations. Answers to the following questions are explored with the parent after the tape has been reviewed:

1. What are the specific areas of competence and the areas that create difficulties?
2. What is the impact of this difficulty on the other partner?
3. Are there specific dynamics of the interaction that need to be addressed, such as turn taking, synchrony, or timing?

After the questions have been answered, interventions can be designed with a specific focus:

1. Targeting the specific behavior of one or the other partner (parent or infant) and trying to change it
2. Targeting the partner's response to the behavior and trying to change it
3. Targeting specific aspects of the interaction for change

Strategies for Adaptations in the Relationship

Stage I: Regulation of Biological Patterns
Major emphasis: Determine whether the child is over- or undersensitive to the environment and help parent to facilitate child's optimum state.

Alerting Commenting and sharing observations: The parent and professional together note whether the infant is passive with low arousal, has a tendency not to make demands of the environment, and/or has muted distress and hunger cues. Conversely, they note if the infant is overly sensitive to outside stimuli with a preponderance of crying

*Table B.3 and the following text are reprinted with permission from MJ Hanson, MS Krentz. Supporting Parent-Child Interactions: A Guide for Early Intervention Program Personnel. San Francisco: University of San Francisco, Department of Special Education, 1986.

behavior, easily shifting states, gaze aversion, and/or an inability to be consoled. Is the parent confused about the infant's signals? Do the partners have very different paces?

Serving as baby's interpreter: Carefully observe the infant's cues and help parents understand the meaning of these cues. Watch for baby's cues that mean "I've had enough" or "I want more."

Guiding   Informing: Discuss how premature birth or disabling conditions can affect state control. Help parents to distinguish different states. Help parents identify engagement cues (cues that begin or maintain an interaction; e.g., looking, smiling, or touching) and disengagement cues (cues that indicate that the baby wants to stop the interaction; e.g., gaze aversion, arching, turning, or crawling away). Help the parent communicate with a "neurologically sensitive" child by using fewer modalities (e.g., using only voice rather than voice, vision, and kinesthetic means). Help parents with a passive child exaggerate their affectual expressions so that the child becomes more interested and alert.

Reframing: Help parents who experience the gaze aversion of their child understand that this is not rejection but an attempt to control an overload of environmental stimuli. Help parents understand that their efforts to feed the child at a fast pace may be motivated by the positive desire to make sure the child has adequate caloric intake and help to decrease the parent's anxiety about this.

Commenting on unique qualities: Help the parents see the child apart from the handicap by mentioning special characteristics or competencies. Help parents to realize the child's uniqueness, such as being sensitive to change in the environment, so that the parents may make additional observations of their own. Comment on the child's qualities to balance the parents' perceptions of the child.

Modeling: Model decreasing stimuli to the "neurologically sensitive" child. Model exaggerated play with the more passive child. Model vocalizing to the child during feedings and play. Model communicating with the child through different modalities.

Experimenting: Try approaching a neurologically sensitive child in a variety of ways.

Highlighting: Comment on the child's positive reactions to the parent. Comment on the parents' sensitivity to the child's cues.

Stage II: The Development of Preferential Attachment Behavior and a Focused Relationship

Major emphasis: Seeing whether both partners are developing an attachment and recognizing ways in which they are forming their relationship.

Alerting   Commenting and sharing observations: Note whether the infant is competent enough to signal attachment and how she or he does it. Observe whether parents respond contingently to the infant.

Serving as baby's interpreter: Comment on the baby's need for specific attachments.

Guiding   Informing: Help the parents know the typical attachment behaviors. Help the parents to know how their child may demonstrate different attachments due to the impairment. Alert parents to baby's withdrawal cues.

Reframing: Interpret baby's protests upon separation as the child's growing attachment to the parent. Interpret separation protest as the indication of a special relationship with the parent.

Commenting on unique qualities: Help the parents to see and accept the divergence between their child's preferential attachment behaviors and what might be more typical. Help the parents understand how they may find it disappointing or difficult if a child cannot show varied or intensive attachment behaviors, such as following or vocalizing, because of the disabling condition. Comment on the more subtle ways the child shows attachment behaviors.

Modeling: Model alternative ways of communicating with the infant, such as through touch or kinesthetically. Model social play with the baby.

Experimenting: See if various physical factors, such as different positioning, visual range, lighting, and so on, can be changed so that they help the baby to be more responsive.

Stage III: Consolidating Positive Interactions and Developing a Communicative Context

Major emphasis: Seeing whether child and parent develop as partners and communicate reciprocally.

Alerting Commenting and sharing observations: Note whether the infant engages in reciprocal behavior. Observe whether the infant responds to gestures and vocalizations and whether the infant initiates these behaviors and then expects a response.

Serving as baby's interpreter: Comment on the baby's attempts to respond reciprocally. Comment on the baby's need for response to their initiations to feel competent.

Guiding Informing: Provide information to the parents about the need for predictability and repetition for a communicative context to be established. Help the parents to see how the child's motor, speech, or cognitive impairments can make it difficult for the child to develop a communicative context. Help the parents find the areas of reciprocal behavior in which the child has the most ease and competence.

Reframing: Help the parents to see the child's initiating behavior and the growing intentionality as indication of a growing sense of self.

Commenting on unique qualities: Note the unique qualities a child brings to the task of communicating or comment on the specific ways a child attempts to respond to the parent. Note the parents' adaptability in communicating with their child.

Modeling: Model extended social play for the parent. Model ways of responding to the baby's initiations. Model turn taking and extending the communication sequence.

Experimenting: Try a range of affective expressions and note the child's responses. Try different paces of interaction with the child to see if the child responds more if more time is given.

Highlighting: Note the development of the relationship and more specifically the growing communication abilities between the partners. Note the most effective ways the baby communicates (vision, vocalizations, or gestures).

Stage IV: Growing Differentiation of the Partners in the Relationship

Major emphasis: Looking for the child's growing sense of self and the parents' encouragement of this.

Alerting Commenting and sharing observations: Note the ways in which the child shows his or her growing independence. Is it across all areas of development (emotionally, cognitively, motorically)? Can the parents facilitate the child's autonomy? How do the parents feel about the child's growing independence?

Serving as baby's interpreter: Comment on the child's autonomy. Interpret the child's attempts to resist the parents as an indicator of the child's growing sense of self. Note the child's need for limits to internalize self-regulatory behavior and to be able to be an effective independent agent.

Guiding Informing: Help the parents identify typical toddler behaviors that indicate the child's growing sense of self. Help parents distinguish the child's emotions as different from their own. Help the parents distinguish appropriate limits for the child. Guide the parents in labeling the child's emotions. Encourage the parents to offer the child appropriate outlets for the child's feelings. Help the parents use verbal means to control their child's behavior.

Reframing: Help parents to see resistant behavior as a sign of the child's autonomy.

Commenting on unique qualities: Help the parents to understand how they feel about the child's independence. Do parents expect too much or too little from the child? Do parents worry about the child's autonomy because of the disabling condition? Comment on child's competence to facilitate the parents' trust in the child.

Modeling: Model appropriate limit setting. Model labeling the child's emotions.

Highlighting: Comment in a positive way on the child's initiative and independent behaviors. Comment on the parents' appreciation of child's growth.

Stage V: Negotiating Separations

Major emphasis: Facilitating and attending to the child's growing ability to function apart from the parents.

Alerting Commenting and sharing observations: Note the times and conditions when the parent and child are separate. Observe the quality of the separation and also the quality of the reunion. Observe the ability of parent and child to communicate from a small distance (e.g., across the room) and observe the modalities (e.g., visually, auditorily) in which they do it.

Guiding Informing: Help the parents use distal communication with a child, such as voice, gesture, and gaze, when across the room to assure the child of their presence. Help the parents to understand the child's "back-and-forth" refueling behavior (e.g., child walks or looks back and forth to the parent). Help the parents to be able to reassure the child from a distance and not just from close proximity. Acknowledge and discuss the parents' fears about areas in which the child does not function well independently.

Reframing: Help the parents to understand any rejection of closeness by the child as the child's attempt to develop mastery and control.

Commenting on unique qualities: Help the parents to understand any areas in which their child may have difficulty with separation. For instance, if the child cannot use a visual modality to check back in on the parent or cannot practice coming and going due to motor limitations.

Modeling: Model distal communicative behaviors for the parents. Model leave taking, while preparing the child for this verbally. Model tolerating the child's frustration.

Experimenting: If separation is difficult, help the parents experiment with leaving the child with a familiar adult for brief periods of time.

Highlighting: Note the importance of the child's separateness. Note the importance of the parents having time for themselves.

A METHOD FOR DESCRIBING INTERACTION STYLES OF HANDICAPPED PRELANGUAGE CHILDREN*

The method developed by Norris and Hoffman (1990) to study adult and infant interaction has clinical application for describing aspects of communicative interaction in young handicapped children who do not yet use oral language. The suggested levels and categories of interaction are useful guides in identifying infant behaviors that have communicative function. They can assist in designing effective intervention strategies based on existing abilities spontaneously demonstrated by the child. The six developmental age levels correspond to the substages of sensorimotor development identified by Piaget.

Infant Scale of Nonverbal Interaction

Levels of Interactive Behavior
- Level I (1- to 3-month rating): These behaviors occur in response to general stimulation and are usually in *reaction* to the adult's actions or the general environment.
- Level II (4- to 6-month rating): These behaviors occur in response to play between people, generally reflecting turn taking but not specific control over others.
- Level III (7- to 9-month rating): These behaviors occur when the infant initiates control in the interaction by imitating actions and reacting as participants share interaction with objects.
- Level IV (10- to 12-month rating): These behaviors include imitations of actual *functional* actions and conventional gestures or vocalizations; their meaning is usually clear in context.
- Level V (13- to 18-month rating): These behaviors are directed at getting the adult to share objects or controlling the game so the adult keeps playing.

*Adapted with permission from JA Norris, PR Hoffman. Comparison of adult-initiated vs. child-initiated interaction styles with handicapped prelanguage children. Lang Speech Hear Schools 1990;1:28, 34–36.

- Level VI (19- to 24-month rating): These behaviors reflect the child's attempts to describe experiences using a combination of short phrases, single words, and jargon; the child often initiates interactions by handing objects to the communication partner.

Categories of Behavior
- Vocalizations, including nonspeech sounds, speech sounds, and words
- Limb actions, including movements and gestures of the hands, arms, legs and feet
- Facial and body postures, including movements of the eyes and mouth and body positioning that are social

Recording Observed Behaviors
The specific type of behavior is recorded according to the following types, listed by developmental level and category.

Level I: 1- to 3-Month Rating
Vocalizations
  Undifferentiated vocalizations done to general environment rather than a specific stimulus
  Generalized squeals or chuckles of pleasure or frustration
  Cooing and other vowel vocalizations produced to general stimuli
  Responding to others' vocalizations with vocalizations in play, not play with objects
Limb actions
  Random body movements showing excitement
  Startle response
  Attracting attention with body movements
  Anticipatory activity (excitement when object seen)
Facial and body postures
  Maintaining eye contact when interacted with
  Smiling or widening eyes when talked to
  Looking at people, not in response to play with objects
  Visually following people and objects

Level II: 4- to 6-Month Rating
Vocalization
  Social vocalization, including vocalizing when action done to infant, squealing when talked to, crying if disrupted, and laughing to interaction
  Vocalizations characterized by intonation changes in cooing; bilabial consonants /p/, /b/, and /m/ produced; repetition of consonant-vowel syllable; and consonants /m/, /b/, /n/, /d/, /g/, /l/, /w/, /h/, /p/, and /t/
  Imitating pitch and loudness changes
  Vocalizing directly to another person
  Vocalizing while playing with toy
  Turn taking in vocalizations

Limb actions
  Social refusals, including pulling away and shaking head
  Reacting to social negatives with cries and frowns
  Wiggling limbs when adult initiates a familiar gesture
  Reaching toward another person or close object
Facial and body postures
  Showing anticipation, including raising arms to be picked up, moving close to
    another, and clinging when held
  Smiling or frowning at other people, but not because of play with objects
  Moving to see what is being shown or looked at
  Joint focus to something presented by adult

Level III: 7- to 9-Month Rating
Vocalizations
  Attempting to imitate speech sounds (may not be same sounds) and consonant
    vowel sequences
  Vocalizations show changes in pitch, quality, intensity, rate, and duration
  Vocalizing to have toy reactivated or adult do action
  Vocalizing at object, then looking to adult and indicating the need for help by a
    pull, grab, and so on
  Imitating nonspeech sounds (e.g., cough, smacking, animals, vehicles)
  Imitating words without attaching meaning
  Babbling phrases with four or more different syllables, including sounds such as
    /t/, /d/, /n/, /w/, /f/, /v/, and /l/
Limb actions
  Imitating movements like waving arm and patting hand on tray
  Pushing away unwanted food, object, or person
  Moving limbs to indicate reactivation or recurrence
  Grabbing adult's fingers, pulling hand, and so on to indicate recurrence
  Performing action for familiar game like pat-a-cake
Facial and body postures
  Smiling and laughing when teased or entertained
  Pulling back or moving to reject something
  Using eye contact to indicate recurrence or help
  Moving by leaning over, moving forward, and so on to follow the actions of
    adults or objects

Level IV: 10- to 12-Month Rating
Vocalizations
  Repeating vocalization if it is responded to
  Fussing, crying, and having tantrums when desired object is removed
  Expressing negative reaction through vocalization
  Using single word to label
  Imitating a series of sounds said by an adult
  Using jargon to toys and people as if talking

Limb actions
   Pointing to noticed objects
   Pointing to parts of objects upon imitation
   Imitating actions that are functional (e.g., eating, washing) or repeating modeled action to make event recur
   Imitating novel gesture
   Extending toy to give without releasing
   Gesturing to represent an action (e.g., wiggling hand to get something to move)
   Using social gestures like waving bye-bye or shaking head no
Facial and body postures
   Wiggling body to continue a movement like bouncing
   Moving body to represent an action (e.g., rocking to represent a rocking toy)

Level V: 13- to 18-Month Rating
Vocalizations
   Using five words
   Using one word for many meanings
   Imitating variety of words
   Using jargon mixed with real words
Limb actions
   Giving object to adult to get toy to (re)activate
   Pointing, reaching, or grabbing objects or toys to indicate wanting them
   Repeating actions that produce laughter or attention
   Using gestures in combination to indicate wants
Facial and body postures
   Imitating facial movement or expression
   Leading adult by hand to desired object

Level VI: 19- to 24-Month Rating
Vocalizations
   Vocabulary of 10–50 words
   Imitating two- and three-word combinations
   Attempting to describe experiences using jargon mixed with real words
   Using a variety of word classes (e.g., actions, agents, attributes)
Limb actions
   Handing book or object to be read or shared
   Doing a series of related actions
Facial and body postures
   Doing own action if other person does not respond

COMMUNICATIVE TEMPTATIONS*

This activity list is designed to optimize the probability of communicative acts on the part of a child, avoiding the common practice of asking the child to name different objects. Depending on the circumstances, the child's caregiver may be instructed to carry out the activities, or the clinician may do so. The clinician observes the child's communicative means and functions as the activities are in progress. A third person can be used to record responses or to videotape the process for later analysis, freeing the clinician to engage in the activity at hand.

1. Display attractive snack food in a clear plastic sandwich bag. Open bag and begin eating without offering the child any. You may offer some to the mother or accompanying adult. Record child's reaction.

2. Inflate a balloon as child watches. Release it suddenly, allowing it to dart about the room erratically. Retrieve it, and hold it in child's view and wait for response.

3. Inflate a balloon, slowly release the air as child watches, holding it within child's view. Observe and record child's response.

4. Activate a wind-up toy and allow it to run down. Wait for child's response without comment or present the toy to the child and indicate that it is his or her turn to play with it.

5. Hand the child four similar or identical objects (e.g., blocks, plastic figures) to drop into a bucket or box. Provide a different item (e.g., small car or cup) to the child on the fifth occasion. Record reaction.

6. Present a toy or edible the child is known to dislike, offering it assertively. Observe response.

7. Demonstrate how a "clicker" toy (e.g., frog or insect replica with a metal lever on the underside) is operated and allow the child to operate it. Replace the toy with an identical one whose clicker is inoperable and encourage the child to make it work. Observe child's response.

8. Place an attractive toy or preferred food item in a clear plastic jar with a tight-fitting lid. Put the jar in front of the child. Observe response.

9. Place a noise-making object in a brown paper bag and put the bag in front of the child. Observe response.

10. Provide the child with materials to engage in an interesting task (e.g., paper and crayon); "sabotage" the activity by "accidentally" tearing the paper or breaking off the point of the crayon. Observe response.

11. Hold (or have a third person hold) two hand puppets under the table surface. Knock on the table and call the puppets, bringing them out on three consecutive occasions as a pair. On the fourth round, have only one appear. Observe response.

12. Look through age-appropriate books with the child, pointing to pictured objects and looking at the child expectantly.

13. Provide child with a woman's purse or zippered bag containing a set of keys, a mirror, a pencil and pad, or other interesting objects the mother may typically carry. Allow the child to play with the purse, assisting in opening it, if necessary. Observe reaction.

14. Using a piece of waxed paper or a tray as a surface, place the child's hands in a sticky, cold, or wet substance, such as whipped cream, gelatin dessert, Play-Doh, flour and water paste, or white glue. Observe response. Note: Have a wet washcloth and dry towel to clean child's hands when finished.

*Adapted with permission from A Wetherby, BM Prizant. The expression of communicative intent: assessment guidelines. Semin Lang 1989;10:77–91; A Wetherby, C Prutting. Profiles of communicative and cognitive social abilities in autistic children. J Speech Hear Res 1984;27:364–377; with supplemental items from Billeaud 1997.

15. Engage the child in an activity that requires use of specific materials (e.g., paper, crayon, scissors, cotton balls, glue); have a third person remove an essential item, taking a seat across the room with the object in plain view of the child. Observe reaction.

16. Provide child with paper and a stapler that is loaded with only a few staples. Show child how to use the device without expending the supply of staples. Allow the child to operate the stapler, observing reaction when staple supply is exhausted.

17. Have two identical colored felt-tip markers on hand, one that is operable and the other dry. Allow the child to mark on paper with the one that works, replacing it with the one that does not. Hold the operable one in the child's view or use it to show the child that you have one that makes marks. Observe child's response.

18. Show the child two toy cars or trucks, one of which has a missing wheel. Allow child to play with the intact toy as you operate the one that is broken. Exchange toys with the child as the "game" progresses. Observe reaction.

19. Provide two balls, one with deflated air, first rolling the intact ball back and forth and then exchanging the deflated one for the original. Observe child's response.

20. Engage the child in assembling a puzzle. After the third piece has been placed, present the child with a piece that does not go with that puzzle. Observe response.

C

Appendix: Administrative References

Table C.1   Directory of Part H/Part C Lead Agencies

State or Territory	Lead Agency	Telephone
Alabama	Education/Rehabilitation Services	(202) 242-9700
Alaska	Health and Social Services/ Division of Public Health	(907) 465-3030
American Samoa	Department of Health	
Arizona	Economic Security/Developmental Disabilities	(602) 542-0419
Arkansas	Human Services/Developmental Disabilities	(501) 682-1001
Native American populations in all states and territories	U.S. Department of the Interior, Bureau of Indian Affairs/ Office of Education	
California	Developmental Services	(916) 654-1897
Colorado	Education	(303) 866-6710
Connecticut	Education	(203) 638-4208
Delaware	Health and Social Services/Mental Retardation	(301) 739-4452
District of Columbia	Commission on Social Services	(202) 727-5930
Florida	Health and Rehabilitation Services	(904) 487-2690
Georgia	Human Resources	(404) 657-2727
Guam	Education	011 (671) 472-8901
Hawaii	Health/Children with Special Needs	(808) 733-9070
Idaho	Health and Welfare	(208) 334-5514
Illinois	Education	(217) 782-4321
Indiana	Mental Health/Bureau of Developmental Disabilities	(317) 232-7842
Iowa	Education	(515) 281-7844
Kansas	Health and Environment	(913) 296-6135
Kentucky	Mental Health/Mental Retardation	(502) 564-7700
Louisiana	Education (Office of Special Education)	(504) 763-3552
Maine	Education/Division of Special Education	(207) 287-5950
Maryland	Governor's Office of Children and Youth	(410) 333-8100

Table C.1 (continued)

Massachusetts	Public Health	(617) 727-5089
Michigan	Education	(800) 327-5966
Minnesota	Education	(612) 296-7032
Mississippi	Health/Bureau of Early Intervention Services	(601) 960-7427
Missouri	Education	(816) 543-4193
Montana	Social and Rehabilitation Services/ Developmental Disabilities	(406) 444-2995
Nebraska	Education/Social Services	(402) 471-2472
Nevada	Human Resources	(702) 687-5982
New Hampshire	Health and Human Services	(603) 271-5122
New Jersey	Health/Special Child Health Services	(609) 777-7734
New Mexico	Health/Developmental Disabilities	(405) 521-3351
New York	Public Health/Early Intervention, Child, and Adolescent Program	(518) 473-7016
North Carolina	Human Resources/Mental Health-Developmental Disabilities	(919) 733-7672
North Dakota	Human Services	(701) 224-2310
Northern Mariana Islands	Education	011 (670) 322-9817
Ohio	Health/Bureau of Early Intervention	(614) 644-8389
Oklahoma	Education/Special Education	(405) 521-3351
Oregon	Education	(503) 378-3598
Palau	Education	
Pennsylvania	Public Welfare/Office of Mental Health/Mental Retardation	(717) 783-8302
Rhode Island	Health	(401) 277-2312
South Carolina	Health and Environmental Control	(803) 737-0395
South Dakota	Education/Special Education	(605) 773-3678
Tennessee	Education/Division of Special Programs	(901) 741-2851
Texas	Interagency Council on Early Childhood Education	(512) 502-4900
Utah	Health/Baby Watch—Early Intervention	(801) 584-8226
Vermont	Education/Special Education	(802) 828-3141
Virgin Islands	Health	(809) 774-6097
Virginia	Mental Health-Mental Retardation Office of Prevention and Children's Resources	(804) 786-1530
Washington	Social and Health Services, Department of Children and Family	(206) 721-4115
West Virginia	Health and Human Resources	(304) 558-0684
Wisconsin	Health and Social Services	(608) 266-9622
Wyoming	Health and Social Services/ Developmental Disabilities	(307) 777-7731

NATIONAL ORGANIZATIONS

The following organizations are resources for answers to specific questions; guidance in obtaining services; and assistance in locating credentialed professionals, information, and printed materials relating to specific conditions.

Alexander Graham Bell Association for the Deaf
3417 Volta Pl. NW
Washington, DC 20007
(202) 337-5520

Alliance of Genetic Support Groups
38th and R Streets NW
Washington, DC 20057
(202) 625-7853

American Academy for Cerebral Palsy and Developmental Medicine
2405 Westwood Ave., Suite 205
P.O. Box 11083
Richmond, VA 23230
(804) 355-0147

American Academy of Pediatrics
141 Point Blvd. NW
P.O. Box 927
Elk Grove Village, IL 60009
(312) 288-5005

American Brittle Bone Association
1256 Merrill Dr.
Marshalton
West Chester, PA 19380
(215) 692-6248

American Cleft Palate Educational Foundation
331 Salk Hall
University of Pittsburgh
Pittsburgh, PA 15261
(412) 681-9620

American Council for the Blind
1010 Vermont Ave. NW, Suite 1000
Washington, DC 20005
(202) 393-3666
(800) 424-8666

American Foundation for Maternal and Child Health
439 E 51st St.
New York, NY 10022
(212) 759-5510

American Occupational Therapy Association
P.O. Box 1726
Rockville, MD 20850-4375
(301) 948-9626

American Physical Therapy Association
1111 North Fairfax St.
Alexandria, VA 22314
(703) 684-2782

American Society for Deaf Children
814 Thayer Ave.
Silver Spring, MD 20910
(301) 585-5400

American Speech-Language-Hearing Association
10801 Rockville Pike
Rockville, MD 20852-3279
(800) 638-8255

American Association for the Care of Children's Health
3615 Wisconsin Ave. NW
Washington, DC 20016
(202) 244-1801

Association for Persons with Severe Handicaps
7010 Roosevelt Way NW
Seattle, WA 98115
(206) 523-8446

Association of Birth Defect Children
3526 Emerywood Ln.
Orlando, FL 32806
(305) 859-2821

Center for Birth Defects Information Services
Dover Medical Building
P.O. Box 1776
Dover, MA 02030
(508) 785-2525

Cornelia de Lange Syndrome Foundation
60 Dyer Ave.
Collingsville, CT 06022
(203) 693-0159

Epilepsy Foundation of America
4351 Garden City Dr., #406
Landover, MD 20785

International Association for Infant Mental Health
Psychology Research Building
Michigan State University
East Lansing, MI 48824-1117

March of Dimes Birth Defects Foundation
1275 Mamoroneck Ave.
White Plains, NY 10603
(914) 428-7100

National Association for Retarded Citizens
2501 Ave. J
Arlington, TX 76006
(817) 640-0204

National Association for Sickle Cell Disease, Inc.
4221 Wilshire Blvd., Suite 360
Los Angeles, CA 90010
(213) 936-7205
(800) 421-8453

National Association for the Visually Handicapped
22 West 21st St., 6th Floor
New York, NY 10010
(212) 889-3141

National Down Syndrome Congress
1800 Dempster St.
Park Ridge, IL 60068-1146
(800) 232-NDSC (6372)

National Down Syndrome Society
141 Fifth Ave.
New York, NY 10010
(212) 460-9330
(800) 221-4602

National Easter Seal Society
2023 West Ogden Ave.
Chicago, IL 06612
(312) 243-8400

National Information Center for Handicapped Children and Youth
P.O. Box 1492
Washington, DC 20013
(703) 522-0870

National Institute of Child Health and Human Development
9000 Rockville Pike, Bldg. 31, Room 2A32
Bethesda, MD 20205
(301) 496-4143

National Neurofibromatosis Foundation
70 W 40th St., 4th Floor
New York, NY 10018
(212) 460-8980

National Organization for Rare Diseases
P.O. Box 8923
New Fairfield, CT 06812
(203) 746-6518

National Retinitis Pigmentosa Foundation
1401 Mount Royal Ave., Fourth Floor
Baltimore, MD 21217
(800) 638-2300

The National Society for Children and Adults with Autism
1234 Massachusetts Ave. NW, Suite 1017
Washington, DC 2005-4599
(202) 783-0125

National Tay-Sachs and Allied Diseases Association
92 Washington Ave.
Cedarhurst, NY 11516
(516) 569-4300

Osteogenesis Imperfecta Foundation, Inc.
P.O. Box 838
Manchester, NH 03105
(516) 325-8992

Parents of Premature and High Risk Infants International, Inc.
33 West 42nd St.
New York, NY 10036
(606) 277-0008

Prader-Willi Syndrome Association
5515 Malibu Dr.
Edina, MN 55436
(612) 933-0113

Sensory Aids Foundation
399 Sherman Ave., Suite 12
Palo Alto, CA 94306
(415) 329-0430

Spina Bifida Association of America
1700 Rockville Pike, Suite 540
Rockville, MD 20852

United Cerebral Palsy Associations
66 E 34th St.
New York, NY 10016
(212) 481-6300

Zero to Three: National Center for Infants, Toddlers and Families
P.O. Box 7270
McLean, VA 22106-7270
(703) 356-8300

INTERNET RESOURCES AND OTHER CONTACTS

American Medical Association
http://www.ama-assn.org/
Sign on at this site and establish a free account, which allows access to the following: search tools, a table of contents, and abstracts for the Journal of the American Medical Association and other medical journals.

Apert Syndrome
http://www.apert.org
This site provides information and links about Apert syndrome.

Centers for Disease Control
http://www.cdc.gov
This is an extensive database on health statistics of every description.

ChildHelp National Hotline
800-4-A-CHILD
This is a 24-hour information line for advice, referrals, and answers to general questions and handling crises.

Cure Autism Now
http://www.canfoundation.org
This site provides links to other autism interest groups and information on research and grants.

Communicative Disorders and Sciences Home Page
http://www.mankato.msus.edu/dept/comdis/kuster2/welcome.html
This is Judith Kuster's home page for audiologists and speech-language pathologists.

Directory of e-mail addresses of speech-language pathologists and audiologists
http://www.mankato.msus.edu/dept/comdis/kuster2/email.html
This is C. Richard Dean's list of e-mail addresses of communicative disorders specialists.

Ear, Nose, and Throat Information Center
http://www.netdoor.com/entinfo
This site contains copies of brochures relating to ear, nose, and throat problems. It is maintained by the Head and Neck Surgical Group.

Down Syndrome Home Page
http://www.nas.com:80/downsyn

Fetal Alcohol Support Network
http://www.acbr.com/fas/fasmenu.htm
This site provides information on fetal alcohol syndrome, fetal alcohol effects, and related fetal alcohol birth defects.

Fetal Alcohol Syndrome Resources and Materials Guide
http://TheArc.org/misc/faslist.html
This is a guide provided by the Association of Retarded Citizens.

Fragile X Research Foundation
http://www.worx.net/fraxa
This home page provides information about fragile X syndrome.

Galaxy
http://galaxy.einet.net/galaxy/Medicine.html
This page is a guide to worldwide services and information. It provides information and links to other sources about genetic counseling and information on neurobiology.

The Hanen Center
http://www.hanen.org
This is the web page of The Hanen Center, an organization funded by the Canadian government and dedicated to assisting parents, early childhood educators, and others to optimize outcomes for children with developmental disabilities and communication problems.

How Can I Help?
http://www.iinet.com.au/~scarffam/cpa.html
This site provides information of interest to friends and families of persons with cerebral palsy.

International Rett Syndrome Association
http://www2.paltech.com/irsa/irsa.htm
This is the home page of the Rett Syndrome Association.

On-Line Mendelian Inheritance in Man
http://www3.ncbi.nlm.nih.gov/Omim/
This site provides continuously updated McKusik catalogs of autosomal dominant, autosomal recessive, and x-linked phenotypes. It contains extensive information on specific syndromes and diseases.

Missouri Technology Center
http://techctr.educ.umkc.edu/
This site provides resources on augmentative and alternative communication.

National Institute on Deafness and Other Communicative Disorders–Hereditary Hearing Impairment Resource Registry
http://www.boystown.org/hhirr
This site provides information and resources about congenital hearing impairments and other communication problems.

National Institutes of Health
http://www.nih.gov
This home page of the National Institutes of Health provides access to research on specific conditions. Use the keyword "childhood" in a general search at this web site.

National Parent Information Network
1-800-533-4135
Access by phone between 8:00 a.m. and 5:00 p.m. weekdays only. This number provides access to the largest parenting database in the nation. Abstracts and information on requested topics are provided free of charge.

Parents Helping Parents
http://www.php.com
This site provides access to information about specific conditions, programs, organizations, and ways to communicate with other families whose children have the same condition.

Prader-Willi Syndrome Association
http://www.athenet.net/~pwsa_usa/index.html
This home page provides information on Prader-Willi syndrome.

Sociological Abstracts, Inc.
http://www.socabs.org
This is a subscription service offered by Sociological Abstracts, Inc. (P.O. Box 22206, San Diego, CA 92192-0206) at a cost of $8.95 per month with on-line enrollment. It offers an extensive speech-language pathology database.

Waisman Center
http://www.waisman.wisc.edu/mrsites.html
This site provides links to web sites relating to developmental disabilities.

Zero to Three
http://www.zerotothree.org
This web site provides access to research and information on cognitive, physical, and social development of infants and toddlers.

Glossary

Abortion Termination of a pregnancy by natural or other means. A *spontaneous abortion* is a miscarriage. An infant born to a mother who has experienced many previous miscarriages, especially if proximal to birth of the index infant, can be at risk for developmental delays.

Acute Having a sudden or unexpected onset, as opposed to being an ongoing or chronic condition.

Additive risk factors Those conditions that, when superimposed on another recognized risk factor, increase the probability that a given individual will experience significant developmental problems; the cumulative effect is likely to be greater than the sum of the potential problems associated with individual risk factors involved.

Adjusted chronological age (ACA) Age a preterm infant would be if he or she had been born at term. The ACA is used in assessing developmental appropriateness of specific skills and milestones at a given point in time. Adjusting chronological age is agreed to be appropriate to 12 months corrected age. Many argue, however, that age adjustments for preterm babies should extend over 24 months to assess the child's development fairly. To compute the ACA, subtract the number of preterm weeks from the actual birth date; the product is the ACA.

Alternative communication Any method of communication designed to take the place of speech (e.g., signing, Rebus symbols, fingerspelling, electronic devices).

Anencephaly Literally "without brain," but more accurately referring to a child with a severely malformed, poorly developed brain; associated with profound retardation.

Anomaly Any abnormality of a physical structure; usually used to imply a bad or unfavorable abnormality.

Anoxia Literally "without oxygen"; the term is often used incorrectly to describe the condition of reduced oxygen supply to the brain (i.e., hypoxia). Prolonged reduction in oxygen supply or literal deprivation of oxygen to the brain can cause brain damage or death.

Apnea A cessation of breathing for more than 15 seconds. The condition is common among premature infants and can lead to hypoxia, anoxia, or death. Some pre-

257

mature infants are issued apnea monitors on discharge from the hospital to reduce the chances of infant mortality.

Applied behavioral analysis (ABA) A highly structured language and behavioral therapy intervention approach based on Skinnerian theory and using extended treatment sessions (up to several hours a day) in which classic stimulus-response-reinforcement procedures are rigidly applied. Some use the term *ABA* when referring to an intervention approach devised by Ivar Lovaas.

Aspiration Introduction of solids or liquids in the respiratory system from the oral or nasal cavities; the condition can lead to infection, hypoxia, anoxia, or death. Meconium aspiration is of concern in newborns. Aspiration of any kind reported in a case history signals the need for follow-up information about the incident.

Assessment A term used in different ways in both professional discussions and legal statutes. In the Individuals with Disabilities Education Act, assessment means the process by which it is determined that a complete evaluation of presenting problems is warranted. Under Part H/Part C, assessment is used to indicate a multidisciplinary process by which the strengths and needs of an eligible child and the family of the eligible child are determined for the purpose of developing an individual family service plan (IFSP); in this case, the diagnosis may actually follow the assessment. Eligibility for services is determined through the evaluation process as defined under Part H/Part C.

Assistive device Any object designed to help an individual compensate for a deficit or disorder; in communicative disorders, the term usually applies to assistive listening devices that help the hearing-impaired cope with the loss of hearing acuity.

Asymmetrical tonic neck reflex (ATN) A normal, primitive reflex pattern in newborns that, if not resolved through maturation, is cause for concern and can indicate significant problems in motor development.

At risk A term indicating that a young child has a greater-than-average chance of having a developmental delay or disorder. The risk can arise from a diagnosed handicapping condition or medical, biological, or environmental factors. Federal legislation (Part H of PL 99-457, PL 102-119, and Part C of PL 205-17) allows states to define and include or exclude certain risk groups as eligible for services under provisions of the law; hence, eligibility varies from state to state for members of specific risk groups.

Atresia An anatomic anomaly characterized by the absence of a biological opening (e.g., atresia of the external auditory meatus or choanal atresia, both of which are related to disorders of communicative development).

Auditory brain stem evoked response (ABER) testing A form of auditory evoked potential response testing in which the neurophysical behavior of the auditory mechanism is measured.

Auditory evoked potential response (AER) The neurophysiologic behavior of the auditory system, which is measured by highly skilled professionals using electrophysiologic devices.

Augmentative communication Any method of communicating that involves use of elements other than speech to facilitate intelligibility of the message, including the use of signs, fingerspelling, communication boards, and electronic augmentative devices.

Autism One of several childhood disorders falling under the broader category of pervasive developmental disorder; a serious, probably lifelong, developmental disorder having its origin before age 3 years and characterized by specific behaviors that meet criteria defined in the current revised edition of the *Diagnostic and Statistical Manual* published by the American Psychiatric Association. The condition affects more boys than girls and occurs in three to four children per 10,000 live births. Communicative impairment is a hallmark feature of the disorder as are certain stereotypic behaviors and tenuous eye contact. Autism is probably genetic in some cases; the cause is unknown in others.

Autistic spectrum disorder A term used to infer varying ranges of behavioral affects or characteristics found among children diagnosed with autism. Children with fewer affects, especially those with more advanced communication skills and social interactions, are likely to have a better prognosis than children who have little or no speech and whose social interactions are profoundly impaired.

Bradycardia Slow heart rate.

Branchial arch disorder Any one of several serious birth defects arising from a disturbance in embryonic development involving the branchial arch structures; such disorders often result in communicative disorders and are identified as specific syndromes (e.g., Turner's syndrome) associated with the particular branchial arch affected.

Bronchopulmonary dysplasia (BPD) Damage to lung tissue frequently associated with prematurity because of the preterm infant's underdeveloped respiratory structures and use of the respirator. When tears or holes appear in the lung tissue, the infant is said to have "blown" a lung. In prematurity, BPD is often associated with intraventricular hemorrhage (IVH); the IVH-BPD combination places an infant at very high risk for communication disorders during the developmental period.

Care plan Any of several plans designed to provide optimal assistance to a given child or family; examples include the nursing care plan, individualized health care plan, individual family service plan, and individual education plan.

Case management Under Part H of PL 99-457, the process of coordinating all services needed to execute the individual family service plan. The term was replaced with *family service coordination* under PL 102-119 of the Individuals with Disabilities Education Act. *Case management* is also a term used by many professionals to relate to direct therapy activities. The manner in which the term is used is important, and the operational definition at any given time should be clearly understood by those who are working with the child and family as there can be legal ramifications involved. Medicaid uses the term *case management* to refer to a specific set of procedures for which providers can charge a fee for services.

Case manager Under Part H of PL 99-457, the designated individual selected from the profession most closely related to the child's disability or handicap who performs the functions of service coordinator; the Individuals with Disabilities Education Act uses the term *family service coordinator* (FSC) in place of *case manager*. Parents cannot serve as their own service coordinator, but they can serve as another family's FSC. Under other standards, the meaning of case manager is considerably different, usually being restricted to discipline-specific services. Because of the legal implications, it is imperative that practitioners understand how the term is being used and what is being assumed when one agrees to take on the role of "case manager" as defined under any legal statute or implementation guideline.

Cerebral palsy A term used to describe a number of permanent neuromotor impairments acquired before the age of 3 years; subcategories of cerebral palsy that describe the type of neuromotor involvement resulting from specific areas of the brain are spasticity, ataxia, athetosis, rigidity, and mixed. Prematurity and birth trauma are commonly cited etiologic factors. Because normal patterns of neuromotor maturation occur over time, it can take up to 2 years to confirm a diagnosis of cerebral palsy. Children with cerebral palsy are at high risk for hearing problems and oral communication difficulties, and many benefit from assistive communication devices.

CHARGE association A collection of physical anomalies that can occur in various combinations and to varying degrees, including coloboma, heart defects, choanal atresia, retarded growth and development, genital hypoplasia, and ear anomalies. Children diagnosed with CHARGE association are at high risk for hearing loss.

Charge nurse The nurse in charge of nursing care in a hospital or health-care unit for a given work shift.

Chromosomal anomaly or disorder Any one of many physical problems arising from too many, too few, misplaced, broken, or malformed chromosomes. Many syndromes are traced to chromosomal anomalies; many involve communicative disorders (see Chapter 3).

Chronic Ongoing or lasting; often used to describe a medical condition associated with communicative impairment (e.g., chronic otitis media).

Complex A collection of features or symptoms that suggest the possibility of a syndrome but lack the complete array of characteristics that would justify diagnosing that syndrome.

Condition A given characteristic or set of characteristics that differentiates a problem from a disease process (e.g., cerebral palsy versus progressive encephalopathy).

Congenital   Present at birth.

Consanguineous   Related by blood through common ancestors.

Consultation   An indirect problem-solving process in which practitioners confer with one or more professional peers, parents, or both for the purpose of bringing their collective expertise to bear on a specific issue or problem.

Continuous positive airway pressure (CPAP)   Method of delivering oxygen via nasal cannula, a procedure commonly used for brief periods of time for infants who require supplementary oxygen; extended use can result in physical damage to the respiratory system if pressure is too high.

Cyanosis   Blue or dusky appearance of the skin caused by lack of oxygen.

Cytomegalovirus (CMV)   A common virus that is detrimental and sometimes lethal to the developing fetus; it can cause birth defects and mental retardation.

Delay   Postponement or extended time needed to accomplish a designated activity or skill.

Developmental delay   Defined in two ways: (1) a significant lag in attaining developmental milestones or skills attributable to known or unknown factors; (2) lifelong deficits or anomalies that require ongoing provision of training to achieve adaptive behaviors and can require ongoing use of equipment or supportive assistance in personal care. It is essential that the professional understand the manner in which the term *developmental delay* is being used. Infant-toddler legislation (Part H of PL 99-457, PL 102-119, and Part C of PL 205-17) allows states to define the term as they wish, and the definition varies significantly from state to state. Families and some professionals use the term to include a functional delay in acquisition of developmental milestones, whereas others use it to define lifelong disabilities.

Developmental disabilities   Conditions that are permanent, have a neurodevelopmental basis, and have an effect on functional abilities in the areas of major life activity including but not limited to receptive and expressive language and mobility; the definition also includes, but is not limited to, cerebral palsy, mental retardation, multiple congenital anomalies, autism, and pervasive developmental disorder of childhood, as well as epilepsy, sensory impairments (deafness and blindness), serious learning disabilities, and hyperactivity with attention deficit disorder. Children who meet the legal definition of *developmentally disabled* are entitled to a number of social, medical, and educational services through publicly funded programs. See definitions included in PL 95-602, The Developmental Disabilities Assistance and Bill of Rights Act.

Diagnosis   In medicine, the act or process of identifying or determining the nature of a disease through examination; also the opinion derived from such examination. In general usage, an analysis of the nature of something or the conclusion reached through such analysis. Also, a precise and detailed description of the characteristics for taxonomic classification. The term is often used by medical and allied health practitioners with the modifiers *descriptive*, *differential*, *definitive*, and *presumptive*. The meaning(s) of the term *diagnosis* should be clearly understood and agreed on by members of multidisciplinary teams who, as a result of their various disciplinary orientations, may use the term differently.

Diagnostic and Statistical Manual (DSM)   A standard reference work published by the American Psychiatric Association containing descriptions of and criteria for labeling specific psychological and psychiatric disorders. The *DSM* is revised on a regular basis; practitioners should use the most recent revision.

Dilantin   A drug commonly prescribed for seizure control; if used in pregnancy, the substance can have deleterious effects on the developing fetus.

Disorder   A problem or difficulty that persists over time. A disorder can be responsive to appropriate therapeutic management either through resolution of the problem or through compensatory adjustment.

Dysfunction   Inefficient operation of an expected function. A dysfunction usually is responsive to appropriate intervention and need not be a permanent condition.

Dysmorphic   Abnormal appearance of physical structure(s).

Dysplasia   Abnormal growth of a physical structure of the body.

Early and Periodic Screening, Diagnosis, and Treatment (EPSDT)   A federally funded program that provides free child-health services to eligible children from birth through 21 years of age.

Education for the Handicapped Act (EHA)   A federal entitlement program (PL 94-142), which established the right to a free, appropriate education in the least-restrictive environment for handicapped students from birth to 21 years of age. It was amended in 1986 to require states to provide educational services to preschool children from 3 to 5 years of age under Part B (previously a state option) and to encourage provision of comprehensive services to handicapped and at-risk infants and toddlers under Part H (which remained a state option under IDEA, the 1991 special education entitlement act).

Efficacy   Documentation or proof that a particular treatment is more beneficial than it is harmful.

Efficiency   Documentation that a particular treatment is effective in terms of expenditure of time, personnel, and money (not to be confused with efficacy [see *efficacy*]).

Eligibility   Meeting specified qualification(s) to receive services under state and federal statutes, rules, and regulations; payment for providing such services hinges on determination of eligibility.

Encephalitis   A viral infection that invades the brain tissue; a serious condition that can result in death or permanent disability.

Encephalocele Opening in the skull through which encased brain matter protrudes.

Encephalopathy A disorder or disease of the brain.

Endotracheal tube (ET) A thin tube inserted into the trachea to deliver oxygen to the lungs.

Environmental risk The presence of family, community, or social conditions that are predictive of negative developmental outcomes for infants and young children.

Epilepsy Any one of a range of seizure activities related to electrophysiologic functions of the brain; see also *seizures*.

Etiology The cause or source of a disease or disorder.

Evaluation See *assessment*.

Extra-corporeal mechanical oxygenation (ECMO) Delivery of oxygen via a heart-lung machine to some infants admitted to the neonatal intensive care unit.

Failure to thrive (FTT) A condition diagnosed in the first 2 years of life when a child's weight drops below the third percentile of growth with no known organic etiology.

Fat pads Extra tissue present in the cheeks of infants born at term and absent in preterm babies, which assist the infant during sucking and feeding; also called *sucking pads*.

Fetal alcohol effects Physical features, behaviors, or both that are associated with maternal use of alcohol during pregnancy; this term is used when fetal alcohol syndrome is not fully in evidence.

Fetal alcohol syndrome (FAS) A set of physical traits and behaviors common to children with a history of prenatal exposure to alcohol. Such children often have limited cognitive abilities, specific communicative and learning disabilities, and characteristic behaviors, as well as physical traits that are indicative of the condition. Velopharyngeal inadequacy, submucous cleft palate, or both are sometimes found in this population.

Focal lesions Pathogenic changes in tissues in a localized area.

Fontanel Any one of several soft spots on the baby's head between the bony plates of the skull. Premature fusion of the bones causes limitation of space for the brain to grow and can result in mental retardation; timing of surgical treatment is crucial to prevention of mental retardation associated with premature closure.

Functional skills Abilities needed to perform activities of daily living.

Gavage feeding Tube feeding using a nasogastric tube leading from the nose or mouth to the esophagus.

Genetic disorder   Any of several disorders arising from autosomal dominant or autosomal recessive inheritance patterns; see also *chromosomal disorder*.

Glabella   A smooth prominence on the frontal bone above the root of the nose; the forward projecting point of the forehead in the midline at the level of the supraorbital ridges.

Glossoptosis   Downward displacement of the tongue.

Gravida   A term used to specify pregnancy; usually modified by a number or description (e.g., *primigravida* for first pregnancy and *gravida 4* for fourth pregnancy).

G-tube   A feeding tube (surgically attached through the abdominal wall to the stomach) that permits the child to receive nourishment when there are problems with swallowing or with certain anatomic structures of the digestive system; also called a *peg*; see also *nasogastric tube*.

Haberman feeder   A specially designed infant feeder for use with cleft palate babies; it can also be appropriate for other infants with feeding and swallowing problems.

Handicap   A condition, often permanent, that interferes with one's ability to perform everyday activities in the customary way; handicaps can be physical, mental, or both.

Human immunodeficiency virus (HIV)   The cause of acquired immunodeficiency syndrome, a disease known to affect the nervous system. Congenital HIV places the infant at risk for many problems, including communicative disorders.

Hydrocephalus   An accumulation of cerebrospinal fluid in the head; if not relieved, the increased pressure on the brain can cause permanent damage resulting in mental retardation. Treatment is often provided in the form of a surgical shunt to divert the excess fluid to the abdominal cavity where it can be eliminated naturally.

Hyperbilirubinemia   Excessive supply of the chemical bilirubin, which if left untreated can cause liver damage and, in extreme cases, brain damage or death; commonly referred to as *jaundice* because of the observable skin or eye tint resulting from the condition.

Hyperextension   Overextension of motor movements; when persistent or aberrant, can indicate a physical condition that interferes with typical development of motor functions.

Hypertelorism   A condition in which there is an abnormally wide distance between the eyes; can reflect a family trait but is often associated with other anomalies, suggesting a syndrome.

Hypertonia   Overly tense body tone; can be a diagnostic sign of motor development problems.

Hypotonia   Floppiness of body tone; can be a diagnostic sign of motor or other developmental problems.

Hypoxia Significant reduction of oxygen to the brain; prolonged oxygen deprivation can cause brain damage; not synonymous with *anoxia.*

Iatrogenic Caused by or from a treatment process (usually an undesirable effect residual to use of a life-saving drug).

Idiopathic toe walking An observable behavior of children without neurologic deficits who persistently walk on their toes over a prolonged period during the preschool years.

Incidence The rate of *new occurrences* of a condition in a population within a specified period of time.

Individual Education Plan (IEP) The plan required for every child served under federal special education legislation.

Individual Family Service Plan (IFSP) The document that outlines services an eligible infant or toddler and family are to receive under provisions of Part H of PL 99-457, PL 102-119, and Part C of PL 105-17. Requirements of the IFSP include a statement of the child's current health status, current levels of functioning in five developmental areas, and strengths and needs; a statement of the family's strengths (resources) and needs (priorities) and the services required to assist the family in enhancing the child's development; expected outcomes; the name of the service coordinator (case manager); timelines for provision of services; sources of payment for designated services; and a transition plan.

Individuals with Disabilities Education Act (IDEA) of 1991 The act and its subsequent revisions mandate a free, appropriate education for persons with a wide range of disabilities from birth through 21 years of age.

International Classification of Diseases (ICD) A standard medical reference published by the American Medical Association and used in health care settings. *ICD* codes often appear on billing slips and are used by insurers in connection with reimbursement schedules; see also *Physicians' Current Procedural Terminology (CPT).*

Intervention A term used to describe the various services that are provided to enhance the development of a handicapped or at-risk child. The term is used differently by members of different professional disciplines (especially by counselors and psychologists who may also work in substance-abuse programs). Practitioners should ensure that they understand the manner in which the term is used by colleagues. *Early intervention* or *developmental intervention* is the preferred term in working with infants and toddlers; however, *early intervention* is also used by practitioners to identify interventions offered on recognition of a problem, which can connote a different time frame than is used by infant-toddler specialists.

Intrauterine Growth Retardation (IUGR) Failure of the fetus to develop appropriate body size, weight, or both during gestation; a condition often associated with developmental delays and disorders.

Intraventricular Hemorrhage (IVH) A condition common to premature infants involving bleeding within the ventricles of the brain. The extent of the bleeding is designated by assignment of a grade: grade I is least extensive, and grade IV is most extensive. Informally referred to as a *bleed*, the condition may resolve itself with no discernible aftereffects. A child with a grade III or grade IV IVH is considered to be at risk for communication (and other developmental) problems that can emerge at a later date.

Intubation Insertion of a tube into the body; endotracheal intubation is the process used to administer certain anesthesias. Repeated or careless intubation can result in damage to the surrounding structures, especially the vocal cords, causing difficulty with phonation.

Jaundice A common condition exhibited by newborns; treated by bilirubin reduction lamps (bililights); see also *hyperbilirubinemia*.

Kernicterus Damage to the nervous system caused by excessive bilirubin in the blood.

Lanugo A covering of fine, downy hair on the fetus; its presence in the newborn is a characteristic of preterm delivery.

Laryngeal hypoplasia Underdevelopment of laryngeal structures; it can have implications for both respiratory function and phonation.

Lead agency The designated state agency responsible for implementation of infant-toddler legislation and coordination of efforts among other state and community agencies and provider groups.

Leukomalacia A serious condition characterized by softening of the white matter of the brain caused by loss of viability and function of the tissue.

Lovaas therapy An intensive program of therapy used with children who are diagnosed with pervasive developmental disorder or autism; see also *applied behavioral analysis*.

Low birth weight (LBW) Variously defined as birth weight of less than 2,500 g, but usually understood to refer to birth weights of less than 1,250 g.

Macrocephaly Head circumference larger than normal for age and body size; it can be a family trait or be indicative of hydrocephalus or other significant medical conditions.

Management A course of intervention or treatment provided to prevent or reduce the effects of a condition; often used interchangeably with *treatment* or *intervention*. Members of multidisciplinary teams should discuss and agree on the use of the terms for purposes of their work with infants, toddlers, and families.

Meconium The waste product material excreted by the fetus; aspiration of meconium is a potentially serious perinatal complication affecting the infant's respiratory system. Infections resulting from meconium aspiration can be lethal.

Infants with this condition may be at risk for future communication and other developmental disorders.

Medicaid   A state-operated, federally funded health program available to infants and toddlers whose parents qualify by income or special circumstance for eligibility.

Meningitis   Inflammation of the meninges (tissue encasement of the brain and spinal column) caused by viral or bacterial infection; it can result in brain damage, blindness, cerebral palsy, seizures, hearing loss, or mental retardation.

Meningocele   Hernial protrusion of the meninges (the three layers of tissue that envelop the brain and spinal cord: dura mater, pia mater, and arachnoid) through a defect in the skull or vertebral column.

Microcephaly   Literally "small head"; can be associated with premature fusion of the bones of the skull, which, if left untreated, can restrict brain growth and result in mental retardation.

Microtia   A craniofacial anomaly in which the structure of the ear(s) is small; often associated with hearing loss.

Monitors   Any of several devices used to measure some aspect of the infant's physiologic status (e.g., oxygen intake, apnea, temperature, respiration, heart rate, intake of liquids, composition of blood gases).

Morbidity   Illness or disease; rate of occurrence of disease in the population.

Moro's reflex   A normal primitive reflex. Failure of resolution through maturation of the central nervous system can have diagnostic implications for motor problems.

Myelination   Formation of an outer sheath as nerve fibers mature. Failure of myelination is associated with developmental delays and disorders.

Myelomeningocele   Hernial protrusion of the cord and its meninges through a defect in the vertebral canal.

Nasogastric (NG) tube   A flexible tube inserted through the nose or mouth and esophagus and used to deliver breast milk or formula to infants who have difficulty swallowing.

Necrosis   Dying off of tissue cells.

Neonatal intensive care unit (NICU)   A specialized hospital nursery facility designed for infants with critical care needs; there are four levels, representing increasing capabilities to handle complex medical care of newborns. Sophistication of equipment and staff increases as the levels increase. Level I must provide adequate staff to resuscitate infants born in the delivery room, stabilize sick infants before transfer to Level II, III, or IV units, continue care for healthy infants until discharge, and continue special care for sick infants transferred from Level II, III, or IV NICUs. Level II must have personnel to provide all services listed for Level I units plus intermediate care for infants born in the hospital's high-risk delivery facilities. Level III must provide personnel to serve normal and high-risk infants, including resuscitation, stabilization, and continuing care for sick infants transferred from Level I and Level II facilities. Level IV units must have facilities and trained staff to perform the most advanced medical and surgical procedures (e.g., organ transplants).

Neonate   Newborn infant through age 28 days.

Neural tube defect   A general term inclusive of myelomeningocele, meningocele, spina bifida, and anencephaly.

Neurodevelopmental treatment (NDT)   See *sensory integration therapy*.

Nonverbal communication   Any form of communication that does not use words.

Norm-referenced scales assessment   Measures that compare a child's performance to that of typical age peers.

Occiput   The back of the head.

Osteogenesis imperfecta   A syndrome in which bones are susceptible to fracture; deafness can be a coexisting condition.

Ototoxin   Any chemical or substance that damages the auditory nerve and consequently has the potential to impair hearing.

Palmar grasp   Immature grasp in which the palm is used, rather than the fingers, to manipulate an object. Persistence of this immature pattern can be indicative of fine-motor impairment in young children.

Patent ductus arteriosus (PDA)   A physical malformation of the heart commonly seen in Down syndrome children.

Penetrance   The degree to which a genetic factor exhibits itself in a given individual; some genetic anomalies are passed from one generation to another with varying degrees of observable effects (varying degrees of penetrance of the trait in question).

Perinatal   Period of time extending from the eighteenth week of gestation to 1 week following delivery.

Phenobarbital   A medication commonly prescribed for control of seizures; if used in pregnancy, can have deleterious effects on the developing fetus.

Phenylketonuria (PKU)   A disorder of metabolism that allows accumulation of excessive phenylalanine in brain tissues, which can lead to mental retardation. Most states require PKU testing of all infants. If present, treatment requires strict control of diet.

Phototherapy   Treatment for jaundice using bright lights informally referred to as bililights.

Physicians' Current Procedural Terminology (CPT)   A publication of the American Medical Association describing and classifying clinical procedures. The reference is widely used by medical records librarians and third-party payers, such as insurance companies and Medicaid. *CPT* codes can be used in conjunction with *ICD* codes; see also *International Classification of Diseases (ICD)*.

Placenta abruptio   Detachment of the placenta before birth; a potential cause of spontaneous abortion (miscarriage), hypoxia, or asphyxia in the infant.

Pneumothorax   Collection of air and gas in the chest cavity, which can result from too much pressure of an oxygen delivery system.

Post-term delivery   Delivery of an infant after the thirty-ninth week of gestation. Post-term babies are at risk for a variety of problems, including language disorders.

Pragmatics   A set of sociolinguistic rules related to language usage within the communicative context (See Rossetti LM. The Rossetti Infant-Toddler Language Scale: Examiner's Manual. East Moline, IL: LinguiSystems, 1990;8–9.) Early infant-caregiver interactions are the foundation for the learning of pragmatic rules used by the culture to which the family belongs.

Prematurity   Delivery of an infant before the thirty-ninth week of gestation. Extreme prematurity, especially if combined with bronchopulmonary dysplasia and grade III or grade IV intraventricular hemorrhage, places the infant at risk for developmental problems, including language disorders.

Preterm   The preferred term among medical practitioners for delivery before the thirty-eighth week of gestation; commonly used by the general public synonymously with *prematurity*.

Prevalence   The total rate or proportion of cases in a population at or during a specific period of time.

Prevention   Any activity conducted for the purpose of avoiding the occurrence of a disease or disorder (primary prevention), eliminating or curing it if present (secondary prevention), or reducing its negative effects through treatment if amelioration of the condition itself is not possible (tertiary prevention).

Primitive reflexes   Motoric responses that develop before birth and persist in infancy. Primitive reflexes are expected to resolve in predictable sequences in favor of voluntary motor control by the end of the first year of life. Persistence of primitive reflexes is a significant diagnostic indicator of developmental problems. Because motor development is intricately interwoven with communicative development, persistent primitive reflexes place infants at risk for communicative delays and disorders.

Prognosis   A statement of the probability for full or partial habilitation or rehabilitation based on the professional's assessment in light of all information at hand.

Prone   Lying on the stomach or abdomen.

Ptosis   A muscular problem in which the eyelid droops; sometimes seen in combination with other craniofacial anomalies associated with developmental delays and disabilities; ptosis can also be a family trait of no particular diagnostic significance.

Public Law 102-119   The 1991 reauthorization of the Education of the Handicapped Act, including Part H, renaming it as *Individuals with Disabilities Education Act (IDEA)*.

Public Law 205-17   The 1997 amendments to IDEA reauthorizing and providing funds for special education; provisions for infant-toddler and family services are contained in Part C of this legislation.

Public Law 94-142   See *Education for the Handicapped Act*; see also *Individuals with Disabilities Education Act*.

Public Law 99-457   The 1986 amendment to PL 94-142 that authorized services to children from 3 to 5 years of age (sec. 619, Part B) and gave states the option of providing services to handicapped and at-risk infants, toddlers, and their families (Part B).

Qualified provider   A term used for service providers on the multidisciplinary assessment team required under Part H regulations. Each state is allowed to identify the training and credentials required of those who are deemed to be qualified providers, but such designation must be in keeping with the "highest entry-level standards" in the state for each discipline. Practitioners in each state should become familiar with their state's definitional requirements.

Respiratory distress syndrome (RDS)   A set of symptoms resulting from oxygen deprivation in the perinatal period; often associated with bronchopulmonary dysplasia.

Retinopathy of prematurity (ROP)   A condition caused by excessive or prolonged use of supplementary oxygen in premature babies during the perinatal period, which adversely affects the infant's retina; associated with reduced visual acuity.

Retrognathia   Small, underdeveloped mandible that is posterior to the normal position in relation to the maxilla; a trait associated with some syndromes or sequences (e.g., Pierre Robin sequence). Retrognathia can involve significant implications for growth of the head and facial structures and for dental development; it can also be a family trait of no particular developmental significance.

Rubella   German measles virus. When contracted in pregnancy, rubella causes severe birth defects, including sensory anomalies, heart problems, mental retardation, and deafness.

Screening   A process (formal or informal) by which individuals requiring further evaluation or assessment are identified from a general population.

Section 619   A "shorthand" reference to a section of the federal statute that ensures early and continuing care and education for developmentally disabled children at no cost to their families; funding for such services is provided to states under block grants.

Seizure   An involuntary lapse of awareness or bodily control resulting from abnormal neural impulses; when used to describe neuromotor aberrations observed in infants and toddlers, seizures can be categorized as idiopathic (peculiar to a given individual and having no easily identified cause), grand mal (involving temporary loss of consciousness along with uncontrolled neuromotor activity), or petit mal (involving a momentary lapse of awareness during which the child may maintain erect body posture and seem to be daydreaming). Spontaneous resolution of seizure activity can occur, but children with seizures are at risk for developmental delays and disorders. Pharmacologic treatment is commonly prescribed for persistent seizure activity and as a preventative measure when a history of seizures is present.

Self-stimulation Any habit of a child, the purpose of which is to provide sensory stimulation or self-calming. Transitory self-stimulation is normal at certain stages of development; unusual, persistent, or excessive forms of self-stimulation (e.g., rocking, arm flapping, spinning) are symptomatic of particular problems, including mental retardation, autism, emotional disorders, and some physical disorders.

Sensorimotor stage developmental A developmental stage defined by Piaget generally inclusive of behaviors characteristic of children between birth and 2 years of age.

Sensory integration therapy A form of therapy based on neurodevelopmental treatment techniques developed by Karl and Berta Bobath for cerebral palsy. The goal of sensory integration therapy is to promote gross motor development in children with impaired neuromotor function. Strategies used in sensory integration therapy have clinical applications in calming some children and making them more receptive to therapies involving instruction and attentional focus. This form of therapy is considered controversial among some early-intervention practitioners.

Sepsis Presence of infection in the blood.

Serologic Relating to the study or measurement of components of serum.

Shunt A surgically inserted tube to divert fluid from one part of the body to another; shunts are often used to relieve pressure on the brain caused by excessive accumulation of cerebrospinal fluid in the cranium.

Skin tags Extra bits of skin (with or without cartilage), often abnormally placed, sometimes seen on the head or neck of a child with developmental anomalies; such tissue often represents abnormal migration of facial structures during the embryonic period and can indicate that other problems also occurred during that stage of development.

Sleep apnea See *apnea*.

Small for gestational age (SGA) An infant of any gestational age whose weight and size are below expectations for its developmental level. Leading causes of SGA include poor maternal nutrition, maternal illness, or maternal substance abuse. SGA babies are at risk for developmental delays.

Soft neurologic signs (SNS) Any neuromotor symptom or physical symptom (or combination thereof) that suggests the possibility of atypical neurologic maturation. One sign, taken alone, sometimes raises concern; several signs taken together always warrant further diagnostic assessment. Some children with learning disabilities exhibit an unusual number of soft signs. Research is presently exploring the implications of such signs regarding predicting the risk for learning disabilities among children who exhibit such characteristics. Examples of SNSs include dysdiadochokinesia, astereogenesis, persistence of primitive reflexes, sensory extinction, and diminished dexterity, as well as unusual patterns of form or growth of the hands, feet, and nails and double hair whorls.

State regulation disorder   A condition that, for a variety of reasons, causes some infants to be unable to adjust physiologic functions such as sleep-wake cycles, level of alertness, or maintenance of body temperature; this difficulty is common in infants suffering from prenatal drug exposure, but can result from other factors.

Stenosis   A narrowing of an anatomic passageway (e.g., stenosis of the larynx, stenosis of the external auditory meatus, stenosis of the esophagus).

Subdural hemorrhage   Intracranial hemorrhage usually resulting from trauma.

Supine   Lying on the back.

Supplementary Security Income (SSI)   Federally funded income support for disabled individuals, including infants and toddlers who meet specific eligibility criteria. Significant changes in eligibility criteria were promulgated in 1996–1997.

Surfactant   A substance used in the perinatal period to treat respiratory problems common to premature infants.

Syndactyly   Webbing between the fingers or toes; a condition common to some syndromes that also involve anomalies of the head and neck (because the timing of development of those structures is concurrent in embryologic formations) and can be associated with communicative disorders in affected children.

Tachycardia   Rapid heart rate.

Technology dependent   A term used to describe infants and toddlers who require special equipment to sustain life or to perform specified functions; see also *monitors*, *augmentative communication*, and *assistive device*.

Telecanthus   Increased distance between the medial canthi (inner corners of the eye), the presence of which can be either a familial trait or a characteristic of a congenital anomaly.

Temperament   Individual differences of behavior styles of a child.

Teratogen   Any agent or factor that produces physical defects in the developing embryo.

Therapeutic positioning   The facilitation of specific functions or activities for a given individual through physical positioning (e.g., seating, propping, lying) that reduces or relieves the body's expenditure of energy in the attempt to maintain balance or posture. Therapeutic positioning is usually designed by a physical or occupational therapist. It is imperative that the speech-language pathologist be aware of the benefits of therapeutic positioning when working with neurologically impaired children.

Therapy   The application of specific techniques designed to provide a cure or diminution of symptoms or effects of a disease, condition, or behavior. Sometimes used as a synonym for *intervention* or *management*. For the sake of effective communication, multidisciplinary team members need to discuss and agree on the terminology to be used with regard to primary, secondary, and tertiary prevention procedures.

TORCH syndrome   Acronym for infections in newborns attributable to any combination of toxoplasmosis, rubella, cytomegalovirus, and herpes virus; TORCH syndrome places a child at risk for hearing loss and language problems.

Toxemia   A condition resulting from the spread of bacterial toxins by the bloodstream. Toxemia of pregnancy results from metabolic disturbances during gestation and can result in preeclampsia, a condition that compromises health of the mother and child during delivery.

Toxin   Any substance (e.g., heavy metals [e.g., lead], bacterial toxins, or chemical toxins [e.g., alcohol or drugs]) ingested or absorbed by the body that produces a "poisonous" effect and, if left untreated, can produce permanent adverse consequences.

Toxoplasmosis   A protozoan disease that can cause lesions of the central nervous system in infants leading to blindness.

Tracheostomy   Surgically created airway that allows a patient to breathe through a hole in the neck. Children with tracheostomies usually cannot approximate their vocal cords for phonation. Permanent damage to the vocal cords can occur if prolonged use of the tracheostomy is required to maintain a patent airway.

Treatment   Any means used to cure, eliminate, or alleviate the effects of a disease or condition; sometimes used synonymously with *therapy, management,* and *intervention.* Agreement on the use of these terms is essential to effective communication among professionals, and understanding their meanings should be a priority for discussion by members of multidisciplinary teams.

Trisomy   An extra chromosome of any pair. A common form of trisomy affecting chromosome 21 is Down syndrome.

Very low birth weight (VLBW)   Birth weight of less than 1,000 g.

WIC   Acronym for Special Supplemental Food Program for Women, Infants, and Children, a federally funded, publicly administered maternal and child health nutrition program designed to enhance the health of women of childbearing age, infants, and young children.

Index

Note: Page numbers followed by f indicate figures; page numbers followed by t indicate tables.